JOY'S
LIFE
DIET

JOY'S LIFE DIET

Four Steps to Thin Forever

Joy Bauer

with Carol Svec

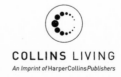

COLLINS LIVING

An Imprint of HarperCollins Publishers

JOY'S LIFE DIET. Copyright © 2009 by Joy Bauer. All rights reserved. Printed in the United States of America. No part of this book may be used or reproduced in any manner whatsoever without written permission except in the case of brief quotations embodied in critical articles and reviews. For information, address HarperCollins Publishers, 10 East 53rd Street, New York, NY 10022.

HarperCollins books may be purchased for educational, business, or sales promotional use. For information, please write: Special Markets Department, HarperCollins Publishers, 10 East 53rd Street, New York, NY 10022.

FIRST EDITION

Designed by Jaime Putorti

Library of Congress Cataloging-in-Publication Data is available upon request.

ISBN 978-0-06-166574-5

09 10 11 12 13   WBC/QW   10 9 8 7 6 5 4 3 2 1

To my LIFElines:
Ian, Jesse, Cole, and Ayden Jane

ACKNOWLEDGMENTS

Many extraordinary people were involved in the creation of this book, and I am deeply and forever grateful. I'm especially thankful to my personal clients and the Joy Fit Club members—their achievements are pure inspiration and their success stories have taught me invaluable weight-loss lessons. Special thanks go to those of you who have publicly shared your journey in this book, and to the countless LIFE dieters who followed the plan before publication and validated that *it works*.

I feel particularly grateful to my good friend Carol Svec—a talented writer who makes my work shine. And, as always, thanks to her husband, Bill, for allowing me to borrow his fabulous wife for months at a time.

Jane Dystel, Miriam Goderich, Lauren Abramo and the rest of the crew at Dystel and Goderich Literary Management are exceptional. It is rare to find such a supportive and accessible team of agents. Thank you!

Gigantic thanks to Susan Turkell, the director of services at Joy Bauer Nutrition, whose enthusiasm, support, and dedication to this project were truly a blessing; and to Johannah McLean, my director of research, who helped every single step of the way—this book substantially benefited from your smarts and commitment. To the talented nutritionists on staff at Joy Bauer Nutrition—Lisa Mandelbaum, Jennifer Medina, Laura Pumillo, Erica Ilton, Elyssa Hurlbut, Nicole Dilorenzo,

Amy Horwitz, Danielle Getty, Laura Wuhl, Ilyse Shapiro, and Suzanne Magnotta—I hope I express my ongoing and daily appreciation for your considerable skills.

Tremendous thanks to the LIFE Diet coaches and recipe testers who were almost as enthusiastic about this project as I was: Alisa Vetter, Amy Horwitz, Carol Bauer, Danielle Getty, Erica Dayan, Dr. Howard Dinowitz, Jen Weingarten, Johannah McLean, Katrina Seidman, Nicole Anziani, Pamela Cole, Susan Turkell, Tara Shokouhi-Razi, Tracy Lockwood, and Wendy Caamano.

The LIFE Diet would not be the same without the contributions of my exercise and food experts. My good friend Geralyn Coopersmith is the outstanding fitness expert who helped me develop a cutting-edge exercise program. And the three phenomenal, health-conscious chefs who helped to create absolutely delicious (and foolproof) recipes are Deborah Gelman, Emily Klein, and Michele Goff.

To everyone at HarperCollins, I offer enthusiastic thanks (to match your enthusiasm) for believing in me and inviting me to be a part of your impressive family. I would like to personally thank my editor and friend, Mary Ellen O'Neill, as well as Michael Morrison, Steve Ross, Margot Schupf, Angie Lee, Shelby Meizlik, Paul Olsewski, Doug Jones, Amy Vreeland, Richard Ljoenes, Matthew Patin, Andrea Rosen, and David Sweeney.

Great big thanks to my friends at the *TODAY Show* who enable me to improve the health of America. You seriously make it a pleasure to work! Heartfelt thanks to Jim Bell, Steve Capus, Phil Griffin, Elena Nachmanoff, Don Nash, Amy Chiaro, Marc Victor, Jaclyn Levin, Brian Balthazar, Rainy Farrell, Amanda Marshall, Jayme Baron, Melanie Jackson, Tammy Filler, Katie Distler, and the countless producers and assistants who help me each week.

Thanks also to the fabulous *TODAY* hosts: Matt Lauer, Meredith Vieira, Ann Curry, Al Roker, Natalie Morales, Hoda Kotb, Kathie Lee Gifford, Amy Robach, and David Gregory. Special thanks to my medical guru, Dr. Nancy Snyderman.

Also, thank goodness for Laura Bonanni-Castorino, Suzie Alvarez, John Digioia, Janet Flora, Mary Kahler, Donna Richards, Joe Tassone, Deb Weber, Keith Shaw, Edward Helbig, April Bartlett, Bianca Henry, Anna Helm, Deb Winson, Paul Giwoyna, Ray Lutz, Susan Houriet, Jen Brown, Rina Raphael and everyone else in the hardworking stage crew, prop department, and wardrobe, hair, makeup, and Web site.

Many thanks to my agents at the William Morris Agency: Brian Dubin, Betsy Berg, Eric Zohn, and Ken Slotnick. And of course, thanks to Ashlea and Suzanne as well. At Waterfront Media, I would like to thank Mike Keriakos, Steven Petrow, Karim Faraq, Roseann Henry, Marianne Goldstein, Dan Wilmer, and Alice Cronin for understanding the magnitude and many dimensions of my LIFE program. And thanks to Ramez Toubassy, Jaime Lewisohn, and the entire Brand Sense company.

Special thanks to Irwin Simon, Ellen Deutsch, Maureen Putman, and the rest of the gang at Hain Celestial for providing the world with healthy, delicious food!

Thanks to Lucy Danziger, Carla Levy, Erin Hobday, and the rest of the talented staff at *Self* magazine.

My deep appreciation also goes to Janice Kaplan, for her kindness and support. It's an honor to be part of your impressive team at *PARADE* magazine.

Thanks to Amy Rosenblum for believing in me and for launching Joy Fit Club on the *TODAY Show,* and to my friend Pam Fink, for the Good Charma karma. Thanks also to the fabulous Suze Orman and Kathy Travis, for their friendship and valuable input.

Hugs to everyone in my wonderful families: the Beal family (Debra, Steve, Ben, Noah, Becca, Chloe, Harvey, and Jenny); the Schloss family (Ellen, Artie, Pam, Dan, Charlie, Cooper, Glenn, Elena, Trey, and Otis); the Bauer family (Carol, Vic, Mary, Nat, Jason, Mia, Annabelle, Harley, and Jimmy); the Cohen/Shapiro family (Nancy, Jon, and Camrin); and Shannon and Shamar Williams.

To my mom and dad, Ellen and Artie Schloss, who always give unwavering support and a soft place to land when I need to escape the cares of the day— thanks and big hugs.

And finally, to my husband, Ian, and my three children, Jesse, Cole, and Ayden Jane—I continue to owe you big-time! Because of you, my world is filled with passion, light, and lots of laughter. You put true LIFE in my heart, and I love you all more each day.

CONTENTS

Introduction: Changing Your LIFE   *1*

1   Step One—*Release*   *15*

2   Step Two—*Relearn*   *73*

3   Step Three—*Reshape*   *149*

4   Step Four—*Reveal*   *231*

5   Recreation—*The LIFE Exercise Program*   *243*

6   *Joy's LIFE Diet FAQs*   *279*

Appendix   *291*

Index   *307*

JOY'S
LIFE
DIET

Changing Your LIFE

Every diet starts with passion for action. It takes time and an ocean of emotional energy to face the reality of excess weight and admit the need for change. Because dieters believe that every encounter with food holds the potential for either accomplishment or diet disaster, they are always alert and on guard. People who have never had to lose weight don't understand how exhausting the process can be. Yes, downright exhausting.

Your search for the right diet brought you here, which means you have already done the initial work. Congratulations—*you have that passion for action!* I believe that if you are going to expend all that energy, you should get something more than broken promises, disappointment, or a temporary drain of water weight. You deserve to get something spectacular for your efforts. Trust me when I tell you that it is possible to transform more than just your waistline—you can lose weight *and* improve nearly every aspect of your life. This is by far the absolute best gift you'll ever give yourself. That's why I created Joy's LIFE Diet.

LIFE stands for **L**ook **I**ncredible, **F**eel **E**xtraordinary.

Isn't that what we all want, what drives our optimism each time we make a New Year's resolution or buy a new swimsuit? Of course it is! Imagine waking up each morning feeling rested and alert, loving the way your body looks, fitting perfectly in all your clothes, and enjoying a steady flow of energy and enthusiasm. If you are willing to invest even a fraction of the energy you've given to all the other diets you've probably already tried, you can *Look Incredible and Feel Extraordinary* every single day. LIFE—it is my personal code, and it can be yours, too.

LIFE Expectations

I know the power of Joy's LIFE Diet firsthand (after all, I eat food, too!) and from an overwhelming amount of positive feedback from countless personal clients. Over the years, the men and women who followed Joy's LIFE Diet principles have collectively dropped more than 250,000 pounds—the heft equivalent of the population of a small town! I also learned the effect weight loss can have from Joy Fit Club members, those determined dieters who—on their own, without my help—took off between 100 and 300 pounds . . . and kept it off. They went from channel surfing to paddling a kayak, running marathons and triathlons, and hiking across Europe. They feel so healthy and energized that they get remarried on a Caribbean beach, play ball with their kids, go back to college, discover hidden talents, and even forge new careers. They have inspired friends and family to lose weight. Don't believe me? You can meet them yourself—scattered throughout this book are twenty profiles of inspiring people (most are Joy Fit Club members) who challenged themselves to change their diets, never expecting that so much of the rest of their lives would end up altered as well.

If all that sounds like a lot to promise, it is. But it's hard to argue with thousands of similar success stories, large and small. The best part is that *you can be one of them.*

Joy's LIFE Diet takes you through your transformation in four easy, spelled-out, mistake-proof steps. In each step, I give you general guidance, specific menus for each day of the week, portion control, and balanced nutrients in the right amounts and combinations to help you look incredible and feel extraordinary. Here's what you can expect, beginning as early as the first week and increasing for as long as you stick with it:

+ Weight loss (of course)
+ Better sleep
+ More energy
+ Strength and stamina
+ Less bloating
+ Greater self-confidence
+ Fewer mood swings
+ Better memory
+ Clearer thinking
+ The ability to move with greater ease
+ Improved relationships with others
+ The experience of waking up with enjoyment and excitement every day

Sounds good, doesn't it? All these goodies don't happen by magic, though. You also have to bring something to the table (both literally and metaphorically).

1. *Change your mind.* It is important that you realize that starting a diet is not a mark of failure, but is in reality a sign that you have already succeeded. It is so easy to fall into the trap of thinking that you are somehow defective for being overweight and that going on a diet says to the world—and to your own inner critic—that you couldn't get this one aspect of your life under control on your own. Although many people begin a diet in desperation when they have "hit rock bottom" in some weight-related way, beginning the LIFE Diet is *not* an act of defeat. It is an act of courage and hopefulness and success! It means you haven't given up on yourself. What could be more positive than that?

2. *Change your eating style.* I'm sure it's obvious that unhealthy habits are not worth keeping, but ditching them can be tricky. Habits are ingrained in the brain. They are familiar and comfortable, and sometimes they serve to make

other people happy. Every family has a set of rituals, recipes, and cooking styles passed down from generation to generation. While these are a part of who you are, you may have to reevaluate and adapt them to twenty-first-century health standards so they work for you and don't continue to translate into extra pounds. Throughout this book, you'll find specific tips on how to make better food choices and how to substitute healthier versions of some of your diet's worst offenders. I also give waistline-friendly recipe makeovers of many family favorites, such as Chicken Parmesan, Turkey Sausage with Sautéed Peppers and Onions, even Creamy Chocolate Pudding.

3. *Change your loyalties.* If you identify with food, separate yourself. You are not an afternoon chocolate bar. You are not a supersized meal. You are not family dinner. Anytime you find yourself defending poor food choices because they are something you "always" do, stop. You are *not* a collection of bad habits. What you are is a person who wants to lose a few pounds and become healthier. That may sound like funny advice, but you will probably run into situations in which food seems to define you. For example, maybe you are the office candy machine because you've got a jar of snacks on your desk. (If you take away the candy, I guarantee your coworkers will notice and ask you what's wrong.) You don't have to remain loyal to who you have always been. There is a new you ready to emerge. Always remember:

> You are more than food.
> You are stronger than a craving.
> You are more complicated than a habit.
> You are more thoughtful than mindless eating.

You are just as successful on day 1 of a diet as you are on day 301—because success is in the doing. With each passing day, you'll look more incredible, and feel even more extraordinary.

Food Choice Basics

I have made it my life's work to make weight loss as easy as possible. With Joy's LIFE Diet, you don't have to think about exactly which foods to eat because my meal plans do it for you. I tell you exactly what to eat (and how much to eat) at every meal for the first six weeks. It's almost as easy as ordering from a menu.

I'm often asked what kind of diet this is, what is the nutritional shorthand— is it low-fat, low-carb, no-meat? Joy's LIFE Diet doesn't conform to that kind of simplification because it contains a rich diversity of foods from all categories. Steps Two, Three, and Four even allow you to have "fun" foods . . . yes, that includes chocolate! Really, it's just good food in the right amounts, with room for snacks and indulgences. So when it comes right down to it, I guess we can call it a no-gimmick, low-fuss diet.

In sweeping general terms, here's what you'll be eating:

Moderate amounts of carbohydrates, which provide energy, fiber, and a ton of vitamins and minerals. The carbs here are mostly from the "high-quality" categories:

+ Foods rich in insoluble fiber, such as high fiber cereal, whole wheat bread and various whole grains, brown rice, all veggies and fruits.
+ Foods rich in soluble fiber, such as oats, beans, sweet potatoes, lentils, and certain vegetables and fruit.

Joy's LIFE Diet isn't "low-fat," but it is low in *toxic* fat. Good fats are an important part of everyone's diet to maintain cell structure and nerve function. However, saturated and trans fats don't work—instead of keeping cells healthy and flexible, these toxic fats promote inflammation and can stiffen cell walls, which interferes with the way they work. Joy's LIFE Diet dramatically reduces the amounts of saturated fats and trans fats in your diet from the most common sources, including whole-fat dairy products (whole milk, cheese, and ice cream), butter, cream, marbled red meat, and anything containing partially hydrogenated oils.

On the other hand, I encourage you to eat moderate amounts of foods rich in the two "good fats": monounsaturated fats, found in olive oils, canola oil, avocado, and nuts; and omega–3 fats, found in fish, canola oil, flaxseeds, and walnuts.

Proteins are the basic building material for all body cells, and we need a steady supply to help us maintain muscles, organs, and bones; keep a strong immune system; and heal damage. Because animal proteins can also contain high amounts of saturated fats, Joy's LIFE Diet contains *lean* proteins only, such as skinless poultry, fish and seafood, lean red meat, eggs (whites only during Step One), low-fat and non-fat dairy, beans, lentils, and soy.

Four Steps to Thin Forever

The foods you eat are only part of my LIFE Diet strategy. The other part involves making the transition from the old you to the new you. No matter how much weight you want to lose, you can accomplish anything in just four steps.

Step One: Release—is a single intensive week of stripping away negative habits.

Step Two: Relearn—is two weeks during which you "reprogram" your appetite and discover the joys of healthy eating.

Step Three: Reshape—lasts until you reach your goal weight. Along the way, you learn how to create physical, psychological, and nutritional wellness.

Step Four: Reveal—is about reveling in your diet success. By the time you reach this step, you will have experienced the full LIFE promise of helping you to Look Incredible and Feel Extraordinary. And because step four is about finding your maintenance groove, once you get here you don't ever have to go back to the old you. Give the big clothes to Goodwill—this weight loss is here to stay.

Secrets for Success

I know you are excited to get started. I'm excited for you! In fact, I want you to have the best possible experience. Here are a few strategies to ease your way:

Acknowledge and avoid your "trigger" foods. Everyone has a few specific foods that are difficult or impossible to resist. These foods trigger uncontrolled eating. I know people who can eat a perfectly healthy diet until they are around their trigger foods, and then they lose all control. Who knows why this happens. It's like a bout of temporary diet insanity. For me, cookies are a trigger food. I know this, so I try to keep them out of the house (or, when I buy cookies for my kids, I only buy the types I like least). Acknowledge your own trigger foods—I'm sure you know what they are. Then . . . avoid them. They are a bad influence on your diet and your health. Don't buy them, don't take a single bite.

Purge or separate out unhealthy foods. As you begin my LIFE Diet, you'll discover which foods are good for you, and which will keep you from your weight-loss goal. If you live alone, or if everyone in your household will be following the diet with you, clean out your refrigerator and pantry. Start with a clean, healthy palette. Stock your kitchen with the good stuff so that everywhere you turn, you are surrounded with encouragement.

Keep "Unlimited Foods" available and ready to eat. On pages 41–42 is a list of the "Unlimited Foods" you can eat whenever you like, as much as you like. But if you don't buy them and make sure they are ready to eat, you may reach for something less healthy when you get hungry. Many of these foods can be purchased in ready-to-eat packages, or can be washed and prepared in advance. Explore some foods that are unfamiliar to you, learn which foods satisfy your snacky taste buds, and keep those foods on hand.

Pre-plan meals. It is easier to make familiar meals than unfamiliar ones. When you come home from a stressful day at work, you will be more likely to stick to my LIFE Diet menu if you plan and shop for all meals at least a day in advance. Make sure all ingredients are on hand and as ready to go as possible. You can pre-chop vegetables and store them in the fridge for a day or two. And—even easier—you can buy frozen chopped vegetables that can be defrosted (and drained) before use. Yes, frozen veggies are just as healthy as fresh, as long as there is no added salt, sugar, cheese, or other additives.

Eat breakfast within 90 minutes of waking, and try not to eat after 9:00 p.m. Food does a whole lot more than just make our stomachs happy. Every time you eat, it sets in motion a cascade of physiological effects, from release of enzymes and hormones to delivery of nutrients wherever they are needed. Your first meal of the day helps to fire up your metabolism and regulate your appetite for the remainder of the day, so it should be eaten relatively close to waking. On the other hand, our bodies naturally wind down at night. As digestion slows, your last meal of the day—even if it is a snack—is more likely to sit in your stomach and affect your sleep. Late-night eating is a common reaction to the day's stress, which almost guarantees over-eating and bingeing. You'll never lose weight that way. I know there are times when late eating is unavoidable, but make that the exception rather than the rule.

I realize that some people have atypical schedules and are therefore unable to eat dinner before 9 p.m. (for example, people who work graveyard shifts or late at night). That's okay. Simply adjust my LIFE guidelines to your personal schedule, no matter what time of the day or night. In other words, eat your three meals and one planned afternoon snack. With those guidelines, you should be eating something every four to five hours. And use the Unlimited List whenever you need it.

Make the TV room a NO EATING ZONE. Too many people indulge in mindless snacking in front of the television, and that's a particularly dangerous habit. It becomes automatic, like buying popcorn at the movies. It doesn't matter what you eat—mindlessly eating even healthy foods can rack up the calories. Try to remain conscious of everything you eat. If you train yourself to eat at the kitchen table, you'll be less susceptible to constant munching. Of course, this assumes that you don't have a television in the kitchen—if you do, keep it turned off while eating.

Motivation Activation

I could give you a million reasons for losing weight; chances are you have heard most of them already. But in the end, one reason stands alone and above them all—the one that brought you to this book. Everyone has a different motivation for beginning a diet. Regardless of whether you want to look slimmer, fit into a different size of clothing, prevent disease, avoid surgery, or be an example to your child, your personal desire and sense of commitment are the only things that will carry you through to achieving permanent weight loss.

I won't lie to you: There will be times when the weight will practically fall off, and times when you will want to pack your bags and move into a Krispy Kreme shop. That happens to everyone. In the tough times, it is important to find a way to remind yourself of your ultimate goal, and that single critical reason that spurred you to start dieting in the first place. Find a way to make it real for yourself, something that you can turn to whenever you need to reactivate your motivation. Some examples that seem to work are:

- ✦ Keep a journal to keep track of your emotional and physical progress.
- ✦ Post a picture of something that reminds you of your weight loss goal—a photo of your child or grandchild, a postcard of the beach where you hope to wear a new swimsuit, a magazine picture of the wedding dress you plan to wear, or anything else that makes your goal a little more concrete.
- ✦ Create a chart or graph that will allow you to visualize your day-to-day weight loss.
- ✦ Create a playlist of songs you find inspirational (and play them often).
- ✦ Find a diet buddy who can relate to your difficulties and be there when you need to have your motivation reenergized. You can find others like you who are following Joy's LIFE Diet at www.JoyBauer.com, where you will also find meal plans, additional recipes, weight loss tools, an interactive weight tracker, an activity calculator, nutrition information, and even an online journal to help keep yourself motivated.

In the coming pages you'll read lots more motivation suggestions in the profiles of real life weight loss superstars. They are here to inspire you! But I also want you to take advantage of your own natural enthusiasm and get started on Joy's LIFE Diet. Right now.

TORY & ROY KLEMENTSEN

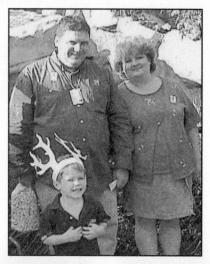

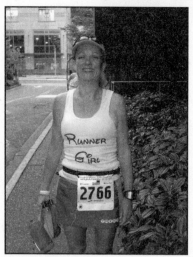

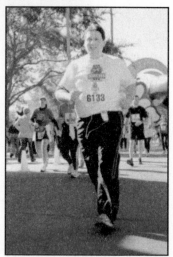

LOST: 204 pounds—102 pounds each!

AGE: both 42

HEIGHT: Tory is 5'3" and Roy is 5'8"

BEFORE: Tory was 222 pounds, size 22/24   Roy was 319 pounds

AFTER: Tory is now 120 pounds, size 2   Roy is now 217 pounds

THIN ACCOMPLISHMENTS: Tory and Roy have run marathons and half marathons. Tory is getting a personal trainer certification.

THIN CHALLENGES:

TORY: Keeping up with wardrobe demands! There were times when I dropped two sizes in a single month. Thank heavens for thrift stores.

ROY: I'm a cheater. I can't go by a fast-food place without stopping by. Now I try to drive roads that avoid the "golden strip" of temptation.

WORDS OF WISDOM:

TORY: How much does your weight add or subtract from your value, truly? When I think back to when I was fat, I'm angry knowing that I wasted so much of my life feeling worthless. I'm healthier now, but I'm the same person I always was.

ROY: KEEP TRYING! Don't give up. If you backslide, start again. I got frustrated often and hit a major plateau. But once I started using Joy Bauer's plan, the plateau broke and the weight came off.

WHAT WAS YOUR TURNING POINT FOR WANTING TO LOSE WEIGHT?

TORY: I was sitting in a mall and saw this gorgeous teenager go skipping by. I said to myself, *I'd do anything to look like that.* And this little voice deep inside me replied: *Yeah, anything but eat right and exercise!* How do you argue with your own little voice?

ROY: I couldn't fit into any of the good rides at Disney World anymore. When you have a hard time fitting into the seat, and the protective bar doesn't come down properly, it is humiliating.

WHAT MADE YOU SUCCESSFUL THIS TIME?

TORY: I was mentally in a better place, not starting from a point of desperation, which is how it always had been previously. You know that moment when you say, oh my God, I look terrible, I've got to lose this weight? That works for a while, but eventually the panic goes away, and so does the diet. This time I built my self-esteem first.

ROY: Tory got me into exercising. Our first day running, we were able to go a quarter of the way around a quarter-mile track. But we kept at it every day. Finally, we did our first mile at our town's Berry Run. We finished, with the worst times of everybody. We didn't care—it was a major accomplishment. And I have to credit Joy Bauer for teaching me the truth about portion control and calories. I thought I would be stuck with those extra pounds, but her program melted them off.

HOW DID YOU BUILD YOUR SELF ESTEEM?

TORY: I stopped all negative self-talk. We beat ourselves up constantly, and that has to stop. The other thing I did was stand in front of a full-length mirror every day—naked. And I made myself say positive things. It was hard in the beginning. I would focus on a part of myself I liked and say something like, well, my eyebrows aren't too bad. Eventually, I realized I wasn't so horrible. It was a slow process, but I learned to love myself from the outside-in.

ON MOTIVATION . . .

TORY: I don't believe in motivation; I believe in commitment. I still love my husband even when he leaves his crusty socks on the floor, but it isn't easy because I'm not *motivated* to love him then. In every diet, eventually the honeymoon is over. I realized I needed to stop depending on a feeling. I was either going to commit to weight loss or not do it at all. Sure, I still have days when I think "this sucks," but I don't let it stop me.

WHAT HASN'T CHANGED?

TORY: My husband, thank goodness. Even now I test him and ask, "Do you think I look better now?" And he always says, "You've always been beautiful to me."

ON THE FUNNY SIDE OF LOSING WEIGHT AS A COUPLE . . .

ROY: Tory dropped weight faster than me in the beginning. She didn't look like the same person, and a couple of people thought I was dating another woman on the side.

JOY'S LESSONS LEARNED

COMMITMENT IS EVERYTHING. *Successful weight loss is largely about attitude. If you want to be like Tory and Roy, make the decision to finally lose all the weight you want and keep it off forever . . . then let yourself become the thin person you were meant to be!*

USE THE BUDDY SYSTEM. *For better or worse, spouses typically adopt each other's habits. If you work together, your weight loss will be for better and better.*

Step One—*Release*

1

love new beginnings, don't you? Everything is fresh, exciting, and bursting with potential. Remember when you were a kid waking up on the first day of summer vacation? Overnight, the whole world changed just a little—breakfast tasted better, your sneakers felt bouncier, your brother was less of a pest, and even the sun seemed to shine a bit brighter. That's the feeling I want you to capture for your first week of Joy's LIFE Diet—that sense of endless possibility and enthusiasm. After all, everything really is about to change for you!

Step One is all about *Release*. First of all, I want you to let go of all your memories of previous diets, of weight loss and weight gain, and any body-related disappointment you've been holding on to. This is a new day, a new program, and your new beginning. During Step One, you will finally be able to break free of food cravings and negative eating patterns. Think of this as a week dedicated to reprogramming your appetite and taming those heavy-snacking demons. And finally—perhaps most important—Step One is about releasing yourself from excess weight. This is the week that gives you a jump start to dropping pounds, purging bloat, and shrinking your waistline. It sets up the good habits, patterns, and skills that you will carry through to the end of the program. Ready? Deep breath . . . now *release*, and trust that you can do this.

Step One is the strictest of all the steps. It lasts just one week—blink and you'll be on to Step Two—but during these first seven power days, you will turn your life around. You'll feel lighter and more energetic, and your clothes (maybe even your sneakers) will begin to fit better as you lose fat and drop water weight. Many people also find that their moods improve, they are able to think more clearly, and they have fewer memory lapses. As you move through each successive step of Joy's LIFE Diet, you'll continue to feel better and better, but this first week is the most important because it holds all your expectations. Think of today as the first day of your adult summer vacation—the sun is up, the world is waiting . . . it's time to jump out of bed and begin your transformation.

JOY'S FOOD FOR THOUGHT

This weight loss program will give you more energy!

Skeptics question how eating *less* food can give a person *more* energy. It may seem counterintuitive, but it's true. When you stick to a weight loss plan, you stop eating a lot of the unnecessary junk food your body does not thrive on. Sugar and excessive fat do a number on your insides by altering your body hormones, which can depress both mood and energy (among other actions). Think of the food changes here as cleaning house—getting rid of the bad stuff and replacing it with the good stuff. You will feel more energetic because you're eating the right food combinations and getting high-quality fuel throughout the day, *and* you'll feel less bloated, sluggish, and lethargic. When the weight starts coming off, you will also feel euphoric. And all this can happen in just a few days! (And by the way, your doctor will appreciate your efforts as your blood sugar, cholesterol, and blood pressure all gradually improve.) That's why this first week of a plan is so empowering—you have the opportunity to see grand improvements on every measure of wellness, including energy levels.

Advice for Success

As you start Joy's LIFE Diet, you are beginning to build a new set of eating habits that will help you maintain your best weight for a lifetime. Soon this style of healthy eating will be entirely comfortable. But until then, I have a few suggestions to increase your chances for weight-loss success.

- ✓ Forget everything you think you know about dieting. I don't want you to worry about counting carbs or calories. Don't compare this diet to other diets you may have tried. Remember, Step One is about release—and that means releasing yourself from all those diets that failed you in the past. Start with a fresh attitude.

- ✓ Eat on a schedule. Try to eat breakfast within the first hour and a half of awakening, and if at all possible, finish eating dinner no later than 9:00 p.m. In between are lunch and one snack, which should allow you to eat something at least every five hours.

- ✓ Pre-plan for your meals. If you get hungry and have not planned ahead for your meals, you are more likely to grab something processed, or sugary, or fatty. None of those things are part of Step One. I recommend going grocery shopping for all the foods you'll need for the coming week's meal plan so you will never be caught unprepared. Also, each night, check your meal plan for the following day so you know what to expect and can prep accordingly.

- ✓ Stock up on "Unlimited" foods. Keep plenty of these safe foods and beverages on hand, ready to grab when you want them.

My Thoughts on Supplements

Eating a wide variety of foods is the best way to get all the necessary vitamins and minerals, and the *only* way to get the many disease-preventing nutrients you can't get in a pill. My meal plans are finely tuned to give you optimal nutrition in weight loss–sized portions. But I understand we all have favorite foods, and there are probably some foods you wouldn't eat even if someone paid you. If you don't consistently eat a variety of healthy foods, consider adding the following supplements to your healthy diet. Because over-the-counter supplements can interact with some medications and are contraindicated for people with some medical conditions, *always speak with your personal physician first before popping anything new.*

Multivitamin: The purpose of a multivitamin is to make up for nutritional weaknesses in your diet. Because vitamin and mineral deficiencies can make you prone to some pretty serious diseases, I think it is better to be safe than sorry. That's why I recommend taking one multivitamin per day simply as an insurance policy. Men and post-menopausal women should look for a brand that does *not* contain iron—they don't need it, and too much iron may result in health problems. Women in their childbearing years should look for a brand that contains 18 milligrams of iron. Choose a brand that contains about 100% of the Daily Value (DV)—the amount scientists have determined is necessary for health—for most nutrients listed on the label. Vitamin D is the exception—optimally you should aim for MORE than 100% DV. Our bodies are capable of making vitamin D, but only when our skin is exposed to direct sunlight. Because of the smart use of sun block to reduce the risk of skin cancer, we are facing a surprise epidemic of vitamin D deficiency. The answer is not to go unprotected in the sun. Instead, be sure to take in 1,000 IU to 2,000 IU vitamin D daily. And the easiest way to get a fair chunk of this amount is with a multivitamin.

There are a lot more options for multivitamins today than there were even just a few years ago. If you can't swallow pills, look for a chewable variety—they make them for adults now, so you don't have to munch on cartoon characters. If your supplement causes you gastrointestinal upset or constipation, try different brands to see if you can find one that doesn't affect you. If all supplements cause problems, stop taking them. Just be extra careful to eat a varied diet.

Calcium with vitamin D3: My meal plans are loaded with calcium, but if your doctor recommends an additional calcium supplement, or if you find yourself skimping on the dairy foods, then by all means take a supplement. Just make sure it also comes packaged with vitamin D3 (cholecalciferol, the most potent form), which enables the calcium to be absorbed. Recent studies suggest that men should not take calcium supplements without the approval of their doctor because of a potential link to prostate cancer.

Omega–3 fish oils: Although it is not absolutely necessary to take an omega–3 fish oil supplement, people who don't eat at least one serving of fish each week probably aren't getting what they need from food alone. Research shows that omega–3 fatty acids play an important role in just about every body system, and the types of omega–3s you get from fish oils are the most potent source. There are two main types of omega–3s from fish oil: EPA (eicosapentaenoic acid) and DHA (docosahexenoic acid). Because fish oil supplements balance these fatty acids differently, read the label and choose a reputable brand that contains at least 650 milligrams of EPA and DHA combined (you'll have to add up the individual milligrams yourself). Note: Avoid taking fish oil in the form of "cod liver oil," which may contain too much vitamin A.

Store fish oil capsules in the refrigerator to keep them from going rancid (and to make them easier to swallow). If taking the capsules makes your breath smell like something that rose from the bottom of the sea, try enteric-coated supplements, which pass through the stomach intact and head directly to the intestines. Always take them with food and plenty of water.

HEALTH FYI

Joy's LIFE Diet is appropriate for people who have type 2 diabetes and/or cardiovascular risk factors. I've made sure to moderate the carbs with each meal and snack. From the cardiovascular perspective, I have included only heart-healthy ingredients to help lower your cholesterol and manage your blood pressure . . . all while losing weight.

Jump in!

Step One sets up the basic structure of Joy LIFE Diet. As you move from step to step, some of the guidelines will change. If you follow the meal plans, you won't have to memorize the list because the rules are built right in.

Step One Food Rules: *Dos and Don'ts*

Joy's LIFE Diet has some very specific rules that help make the diet work. For optimal weight loss, follow the "dos" as closely as the "don'ts." First, the don'ts:

✗ 1. **DON'T** . . . add sugar or other natural sweeteners (including honey) to anything.

✗ 2. **DON'T** . . . use artificial sweeteners.

✗ 3. **DON'T** . . . drink "diet" beverages with artificial sweeteners.

✗ 4. **DON'T** . . . eat processed foods.

✗ 5. **DON'T** . . . add salt to anything.

✗ 6. **DON'T** . . . drink alcohol.

✗ 7. **DON'T** . . . eat any foods that are not on the "Allowed" list.

✗ 8. **DON'T** . . . eat starches during or after dinner.

Now, the dos:

✓ 1. **DO** . . . eat on a schedule and enjoy three meals and your afternoon snack each day.

✓ 2. **DO** . . . drink lots of water throughout the day, including two 8-ounce glasses *before* lunch and two 8-ounce glasses *before* dinner. (These before-meal waters should be consumed up to 30 minutes before eating.) Enjoy as much additional water as you want during meals and throughout the day.

✓ 3. **DO** . . . begin dinner with *LIFE* Dinner Salad or *LIFE* Veggie Soup (see recipes on page 63).

✓ 4. **DO** . . . indulge in foods on the Unlimited Foods List (on pages 41–42). You can enjoy these foods in unlimited quantities at any time throughout the day, particularly when you get hungry between designated meal and snack times.

✓ 5. **DO** . . . feel free to swap meals or ingredients from within the same categories.

✓ 6. **DO** . . . enjoy meals listed in *LIFE* Restaurant Options when dining out.

✓ 7. **DO** . . . feel free to repeat a favorite meal or recipe during the week, as many times as you like.

✓ 8. **DO** . . . engage in at least thirty minutes of exercise every day for the next seven days (see page 260 for Step One exercise guidelines).

step one

BREAKFAST

+

LUNCH

▶ 2 glasses water prior to eating your lunch

+

AFTERNOON SNACK

+

DINNER

▶ Two glasses of water prior to eating your dinner

▶ Always begin dinner with either *LIFE* salad or *LIFE* soup

▶ No starch

SPECIAL NOTES

▶ Enjoy foods from the Unlimited List any time throughout the day.

▶ All men and active women may eat unlimited protein portions at meals only.

in a nutshell

You may be wondering why the *no starch with dinner* rule exists. Although many starches are very healthy and generally good for you, starches are also calorie-dense compared with non-starchy vegetables. And because starches taste good and have a lovely smooth texture in the mouth, we tend to overeat them. That's why I ban starches at dinner during Step One. This strategy has been extremely successful with thousands of my personal clients. I know that it works. Some common starches include rice, pasta, bread, cereals, barley, buckwheat, bulgur, quinoa, potatoes (white and sweet), yams, peas, black-eyed peas, corn, parsnips, yucca, taro, plantains, lentils, chickpeas (garbanzo beans), fava beans, lima beans, and the rest of the starchy beans (pinto, black, kidney, white, pink, red, broad, butter, Great Northern, cannellini, and soy).

JOY'S FOOD FOR THOUGHT

About alcohol . . .

Although many doctors are now "prescribing" a daily glass of red wine for heart health, when it comes to weight loss, alcohol can be a sneaky saboteur. Alcohol lowers inhibitions, which could encourage you to push the boundaries of your meal plan. That's a tactful way of saying that you'll be more likely to overeat or give in to the temptation of a cupcake. Alcohol itself adds calories. One light beer contains the lowest number of calories (100), and the numbers just go up from there. A regular beer contains 150 calories, an appletini and most other martini variations contain about 250 calories, and a large frozen margarita can contain up to 900 calories. Alcohol is off limits for Step One, but you will have a chance to choose it as one of your *LIFE* Healthy Extras later in the program.

Artificial sweeteners and diet soft drinks probably seem like a diet no-brainer, and yet they are on the list of foods to avoid during Step One. My reasoning can be found in the goal of this step: releasing destructive food habits. Artificially sweetened foods may not have the calories of sugar-sweetened foods, but they keep sweetness on our taste buds and our minds. You can't be free of a compulsion to eat sweet foods if you are constantly reminded of the sweetness. This cold-turkey approach to breaking the soda/candy/cookie habit may feel harsh, particularly if you have a sweet tooth, but it is the best way to purge unhealthy habits and move forward with a clean palate.

DEVYN COOK

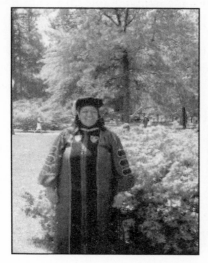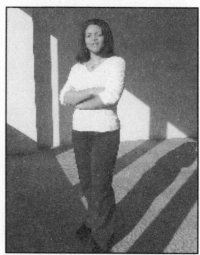

LOST: **167 pounds!**

AGE: **29**

HEIGHT: **5'5"**

BEFORE: **331 pounds, size 28**

AFTER: **164 pounds, size 8**

———————— ◆ ————————

THIN ACCOMPLISHMENTS: Running! I remember thinking that it would be great if I could run a single mile without "dying." Today I ran ten miles, and I'm running a half-marathon soon. I never thought I could do it . . . and I never thought I would like it.

THIN CHALLENGES: I have a lot of trigger foods—bread, cookies, ice cream, chips. I try not to bring them into my house—once they are there, they will be gone within a day.

WORDS OF WISDOM: Try not to put a timeline on your weight loss. I'm glad no one told me when I began that it would take me three years to lose it all because I'm not sure I would have stuck with it.

I was working at Lane Bryant, a clothing store for plus-sized women. One day I tried on the largest sized pants they carried, and I had trouble fitting into them. That was terrifying. I knew I was heavy, but this was a whole new level of heavy. I went out the next day and joined a gym.

WAS IT DIFFICULT TO BEGIN EXERCISING?

It was a big shift for me, but now I love it. I started by walking on the treadmill. Then I started running. At first I would walk ten minutes, then jog for a minute. Gradually, I increased the amount of time I would run. The first time I ran outside was during the Thanksgiving holiday of 2006. I had always seen people running outside and in the parks, and I thought to myself, "Hey, I'm one of them now!" I also tried rollerblading, and recently I started kickboxing with a personal trainer. It's all so exhilarating. I don't think I could have done any of that before.

ON FINDING MOTIVATION . . .

When I got frustrated or discouraged, I would make a list of things that I could do that I couldn't do before. Like running to catch a train or bus, or being able to walk through a turnstile without having to turn sideways. I can look at the list and see how far I've come. That helps a lot. Those little things add up. People who have been skinny their whole lives take this stuff for granted.

JOY'S LESSONS LEARNED

AVOID TRIGGER FOODS. *These are the foods that once you start eating, you simply cannot stop. Common triggers include ice cream, potato chips, dry cereal, and peanut butter. Stay away from your personal problematic foods, whatever they may be. Keep them out of the house. Do not even have one bite. Seriously.*

Step One Foods
Allowed At Meals
(Breakfast, Lunch, and Dinner)

These are foods you'll find in your 7-day Step One menu plan (plus much more). Use this list to swap/substitute foods you don't like within the menus. For example, you may substitute an equivalent portion of an approved meat or protein from the list for that listed at any meal. Let's say you've had your fill of chicken and can't face eating it in your Caesar salad on Day 2, feel free to substitute an equivalent portion of salmon or shrimp. If you're not in the mood for grilled fish on Day 6, you may want to substitute pork tenderloin. Similarly, feel free to exchange or add any and all non-starchy vegetables listed in the meal plan. For example, Day 2 dinner calls for sautéed spinach, but you can just as easily substitute steamed broccoli, stewed tomatoes, or grilled asparagus. ALWAYS remember to stick with the same designated portions.

You may also swap entire meals. For example, if your lunch menu on Day 3 calls for Turkey Burger on Greens but you prefer to eat the Tuna Salad with Pita listed on Day 5, that's fine. If your dinner on Day 6 calls for Grilled Salmon but you prefer the Grilled Chicken Parmesan listed on Day 5, that's fine too. If you don't like the afternoon snack listed on a certain day, feel free to enjoy another one from my snack list. This means that if you enjoy repetition, or if you like to prepare large batches of food to eat throughout the week, that's perfectly okay. You may repeat a menu or meal as many times during the week as you like. If you like Monday's breakfast, you may have the same breakfast for all seven days. All breakfasts are interchangeable, all lunches are interchangeable, and all dinners are interchangeable. But you *can't* eat a dinner for breakfast, or vice versa. Keep repetitions within the same meal category.

There are also foods that you can eat anytime, anywhere, in any amount. I've listed these separately on the "Unlimited Food/Beverage List." These are healthy foods that are low in calories, low in starch, low in natural sugars, and won't threaten your weight loss goals. From what my clients tell me, you will learn to love these foods, even if they aren't exactly your favorites right now. Plus, they give you much more freedom in your meal planning. For example, instead of deciding between sautéed spinach, steamed broccoli, stewed tomatoes, and grilled asparagus, you can eat them all, *in addition to* all the other foods included in the meal. This is the beauty of "unlimited" foods.

In later chapters, I'll discuss how to make good choices during celebrations and holidays when large quantities of food have been known to mysteriously appear on unsuspecting plates (or is that just my family?). But now I don't want to make you wait any longer. Let's get started!

Foods Allowed at Meals

(Wallet-sized, printable lists of allowed foods for each step are available at www .JoyBauer.com.)

Meats

Lean cuts only:
+ Bottom round
+ Buffalo
+ Filet mignon
+ Flank
+ London broil
+ Sirloin
+ Top round
+ Veal
+ Venison

Poultry (skinless only)

+ Chicken breast
+ Chicken breast, ground (at least 90% lean)

- ✦ Chicken thigh
- ✦ Cornish hen
- ✦ Ostrich
- ✦ Turkey breast
- ✦ Turkey burger (lean)
- ✦ Turkey thigh
- ✦ Turkey, ground (at least 90% lean)

Pork

- ✦ Pork tenderloin

Fish and seafood

- ✦ Anchovies
- ✦ Catfish
- ✦ Clams
- ✦ Cod
- ✦ Crab (fresh or canned)
- ✦ Flounder
- ✦ Haddock
- ✦ Halibut
- ✦ Lobster
- ✦ Mackerel (Atlantic only, not king)
- ✦ Mahi mahi
- ✦ Mussels
- ✦ Oysters
- ✦ Red snapper
- ✦ Salmon, wild (fresh and canned)
- ✦ Sardines
- ✦ Scallops
- ✦ Shrimp
- ✦ Sole

- ✦ Tilapia
- ✦ Trout
- ✦ Tuna (canned light in water)
- ✦ Whitefish

Eggs

- ✦ Egg whites
- ✦ Egg substitute

Vegan Proteins

- ✦ Soy milk (low-fat/light)
- ✦ Soy yogurt (nonfat and low-fat)
- ✦ Tempeh
- ✦ Tofu
- ✦ Vegan cheese (nonfat and low-fat)
- ✦ Veggie burgers
- ✦ Wheat gluten/seitan

Dairy

- ✦ Cheese, fat-free (all varieties)
- ✦ Cheese, reduced-fat (all varieties)
- ✦ Cheese, Parmesan
- ✦ Cheese, Romano
- ✦ Greek yogurt (nonfat)
- ✦ Yogurt, nonfat plain and vanilla (no artificial sweetener)

Vegetables (non-starchy only)

- ✦ Artichokes and artichoke hearts
- ✦ Asparagus

- ✦ Beans, non-starchy: green, yellow, Italian, and wax
- ✦ Beets
- ✦ Bok choy (Chinese cabbage)
- ✦ Broccoli
- ✦ Broccoli rabe
- ✦ Broccolini
- ✦ Brussels sprouts
- ✦ Cabbage
- ✦ Carrots
- ✦ Cauliflower
- ✦ Celery
- ✦ Dark green leafy vegetables:
  - ✦ Beet greens
  - ✦ Collard greens
  - ✦ Dandelion greens
  - ✦ Kale
  - ✦ Mustard greens
  - ✦ Spinach
  - ✦ Swiss chard
  - ✦ Turnip greens
- ✦ Eggplant
- ✦ Fennel
- ✦ Garlic
- ✦ Green onions (scallions)
- ✦ Jicama
- ✦ Leeks
- ✦ Lettuce:
  - ✦ Arugula
  - ✦ Endive
  - ✦ Escarole
  - ✦ Iceberg
  - ✦ Mixed greens/salad blends
  - ✦ Romaine

- Mixed vegetable blends without corn, starchy beans, peas, pasta, or any kind of sauce
- Mushrooms
- Okra
- Onion
- Peppers (all varieties)
- Pickles
- Pumpkin (fresh, frozen/canned—must say "100% pure pumpkin," no sugar added)
- Radicchio
- Radishes
- Red peppers, roasted (if packed in oil, pat dry)
- Rhubarb
- Sea vegetables (nori, etc.)
- Shallot
- Snow peas
- Spaghetti squash
- Sprouts (all varieties)
- Summer (yellow) squash
- Tomato
- Water chestnuts
- Watercress
- Zucchini

Whole Grains

Whole grains are incorporated into Step One menus *only* within specific breakfast and lunch recipes, and some afternoon snack options. Eat whole grain items only when designated at a particular meal—and carefully check portions.

- Mini whole wheat pita bread (no more than 70 calories)
- Reduced calorie whole wheat bread (no more than 45 calories per slice)
- Rice cakes (stick with plain, 45 calories per rice cake)

+ Wheat germ
+ Whole grain bread (any brand that lists "whole wheat" as first ingredient)
+ Whole grain cereal (any brand 150 calories or less per 1 cup serving; no more than 8 grams sugar; at least 3 grams fiber)
+ Whole grain oats (plain flavor only; traditional, quick cooking, or steel cut oats)

Fruit

Fruit is incorporated into Step One menus *only* within specific breakfast, lunch, and dinner recipes, and some afternoon snack options. Eat fruit only when designated for a particular meal. Make careful note to only eat the amount listed—some meals list "HALF servings" and others list "WHOLE servings." (Note: When making substitutions, just be sure to pick from the right serving size.)

HALF Fruit Serving Options
+ Apple: 1 small (palm-sized)
+ Apricot: 6 dried halves, or 3 (fresh or dried) whole
+ Banana: ½ medium
+ Berries: ¾ cup (fresh or frozen, unsweetened blueberries, raspberries, blackberries, boysenberries, or sliced strawberries; or 10 whole strawberries)
+ Cantaloupe: ¼ medium or 1 cup cubed
+ Cherries (fresh): ½ cup (about 10 whole)
+ Clementines: 2
+ Fruit salad: ½ cup fresh cut (from the produce section, unsweetened)
+ Grapefruit: ½ (red, pink, or white)
+ Grapes (seedless): ½ cup (red, purple, green, or black)
+ Honeydew melon: 1 cup cubed
+ Kiwi: 1 whole
+ Mango: ½ fresh or ½ cup chunks (unsweetened)
+ Nectarine: 1 whole
+ Orange: 1 medium
+ Papaya (fresh): 1 cup cubed

- Peach: 1 whole
- Pear: ½ large or 1 small
- Pineapple chunks (fresh): ½ cup
- Plum: 1 large
- Pomegranate: ½ medium
- Prunes: 3
- Raisins: 2 tablespoons
- Tangerine: 1 whole
- Watermelon: 1 cup cubed

WHOLE Fruit Serving Options

- Apple: 1 large
- Apricot: 12 dried halves, or 6 (dried or fresh) whole
- Banana: 1 whole
- Berries: 1½ cups (fresh or frozen, unsweetened blueberries, raspberries, blackberries, boysenberries, or sliced strawberries; or 20 whole strawberries)
- Cantaloupe: ½ medium or 2 cups cubed
- Cherries (fresh): 1 cup (about 20 whole)
- Clementines: 3
- Fruit salad: 1 cup fresh cut (from the produce section, unsweetened)
- Grapefruit: 1 whole (red, pink, or white)
- Grapes (seedless): 1 cup (red, purple, green, or black)
- Honeydew melon: 2 cups cubed
- Kiwi: 2 large
- Mango: 1 medium fresh or 1 cup chunks (unsweetened)
- Nectarines: 2
- Oranges: 2 medium
- Papaya (fresh): 2 cups cubed
- Peaches: 2 large
- Pear: 1 large
- Pineapple chunks: 1 cup fresh
- Plums: 2 large
- Pomegranate: 1 medium

- ✦ Prunes: 6
- ✦ Raisins: ¼ cup
- ✦ Tangerines: 2
- ✦ Watermelon: 2 cups cubed

FRUIT OFF SEASON

Many of the meals included in Step One include fresh berries as a fruit option. Out-of-season berries are often underripe, not to mention quite expensive. If you're craving blueberries, strawberries, blackberries, or raspberries in the dead of winter, look for bagged, frozen varieties in your local grocery store. Frozen berries are nearly equivalent to fresh in terms of nutrient content and can be significantly cheaper and tastier during winter months. Just make sure the package doesn't contain any syrup, sugar, or other additives that add unnecessary calories. Measure out the serving size listed in your meal plan while the berries are still frozen (before any settling occurs) and store the rest in the freezer. Then, simply defrost in the microwave or thaw in the refrigerator overnight. Some stores even carry frozen peach slices or mango chunks, so be sure to take advantage of these convenient products to spice up your fruit intake.

Seasonings, Condiments, Marinades, and Healthy Fats

Your meal plans for Step One make use of the following ingredients to flavor and jazz up your meals. Some of the condiments, such as vinegar, mustard, and hot sauce, are also included on the Unlimited List (see pages 41–42) and therefore can be added in unlimited quantities to ANY meal or snack, whether specified or not. For items not found on the Unlimited List, such as ketchup, mayo, and salad dressings, always stick with the portions designated in your meal plan.

- Avocado
- Chiles or hot peppers, fresh or canned in vinegar/water
- Extracts (vanilla, almond, peppermint, etc.)
- Horseradish
- Hot sauce
- Ketchup
- Lemon, fresh
- Lime, fresh
- Marinara sauce (opt for brands with 60 calories or less per half cup serving)
- Mayo, reduced-fat (any brand, 25 calories or less per tablespoon)
- Mustard (plain, brown, spicy, Dijon)
- Nonstick cooking spray (any variety)
- Nuts (almonds, pistachios, walnuts, etc.)
- Nut butters (peanut, soy, almond, etc.)
- Olive oil
- Salad dressing, Caesar (only use for Caesar salad lunch option—any brand, no more than 80 calories per 2 tablespoons)
- Salad dressing, low-calorie (any brand with no more than 40 calories per 2 tablespoons)
- Salad dressing, any of Joy's *LIFE* recipes (pages 60–63)
- Salsa (mild or spicy; any brand without added sugar or corn syrup)
- Salt substitute
- Soy sauce, low-sodium
- Teriyaki sauce, low-sodium
- Vinegar, any type—not vinaigrette
- Wasabi
- Herbs and Spices
    - Allspice
    - Anise seed
    - Basil
    - Bay leaves
    - Cardamom
    - Cayenne pepper

- Celery seed
- Chili powder
- Chinese five-spice
- Chives
- Cilantro
- Cinnamon
- Cloves
- Coriander
- Cumin
- Curry powder
- Dill weed
- Garlic powder
- Ginger
- Lemongrass
- Marjoram
- Mint
- Mustard
- Mustard seed
- Nutmeg
- Old Bay seasoning
- Onion powder
- Oregano
- Paprika
- Parsley
- Pepper (ground) and whole peppercorns
- Pumpkin pie spice
- Red pepper flakes
- Rosemary
- Sage
- Seasoning blends (without added sugar or salt)
- Tarragon
- Thyme
- Turmeric

NATURALLY FLAVORED ZERO-CALORIE COFFEES

Here are two ways to get a flavor boost in your coffee.

1. Add one of the following to your coffee filter basket before brewing (per 6- to 8-cup pot of coffee):

Cinnamon coffee: 1 teaspoon cinnamon

Nutmeg coffee: ½ teaspoon nutmeg

Autumn Harvest coffee: 1 teaspoon pumpkin pie spice

2. Mix one of the following into a brewed pot of coffee (per 6 to 8 cups coffee):

Vanilla coffee: 1 teaspoon vanilla extract

Almond coffee: ¼ teaspoon almond extract

Beverages

- Club soda
- Coffee (no artificial sweeteners or natural sweeteners, including sugar. No cream or whole milk. You may add skim, 1%, or low-fat soy milk only.)
- Naturally flavored zero-calorie coffee with no natural or artificial sweeteners
- Seltzer, zero calorie (plain and naturally flavored)
- Sparkling water
- Tea—black, white, green, herbal (no artificial sweeteners or natural sweeteners, including sugar or honey
- Water
- Naturally flavored waters, calorie-free

CALORIE-FREE, NATURALLY FLAVORED WATERS

These flavored waters are so simple that you may be surprised by how refreshing and satisfying they are.

Start with a glass of cold or sparkling water and add one of the following combos:

Slice of lemon and sprig of thyme

Slice of lemon and sprig of rosemary

Slice of cucumber and several bruised fresh mint leaves

Slice of orange and slice of lime

Slice of lime and several bruised fresh mint leaves

2 sliced strawberries and several bruised fresh mint leaves

Slice of grapefruit and 1 bruised/crushed stalk lemongrass

Slice of grapefruit and 1 sprig rosemary

Acceptable Mid-Afternoon Snack List

You may substitute afternoon snacks listed on your menu with the following options. Stick with one per day, and pay close attention to designated portions.

Cheese Options

+ 1 ounce reduced-fat or fat-free cheese with unlimited celery and pepper sticks
+ 1 ounce reduced-fat or fat-free cheese with 1 mini whole-grain pita (no more than 70 calories) or rice cake
+ 1 ounce reduced-fat or fat-free cheese with 10 raw almonds or 15 pistachio nuts
+ 1 part-skim cheese stick with a HALF fruit serving (see list)

- ✦ 4 level tablespoons reduced-fat or fat-free cream cheese with unlimited celery sticks
- ✦ ½ cup low-fat or nonfat cottage cheese, topped with a HALF fruit serving
- ✦ ½ cup low-fat or nonfat cottage cheese with unlimited nonstarchy vegetables (i.e., cherry tomatoes, red pepper strips, celery, or baby carrots)
- ✦ ¾ cup low-fat or nonfat cottage cheese, plain or with cinnamon
- ✦ 1 slice reduced calorie, whole-grain toast (any brand, 45 calories or less per slice) with 1 ounce slice reduced or nonfat cheese and optional tomato slices
- ✦ 1 slice reduced calorie, whole-grain toast (any brand, 45 calories or less per slice) with 1 level tablespoon reduced-fat or fat-free cream cheese

Yogurt Options

- ✦ 8 ounces nonfat plain, Greek, or vanilla yogurt (no artificial sweeteners)
- ✦ 6 ounces nonfat plain or Greek yogurt (no artificial sweeteners), topped with 2 tablespoons wheat germ or ground flaxseed
- ✦ 6 ounces nonfat plain or Greek yogurt (no artificial sweeteners), topped with a HALF fruit serving

Nut and Nut Butter Options

- ✦ 10 raw almonds or 15 pistachios and a HALF fruit serving
- ✦ 10 raw almonds or 15 pistachios and ½ cup (one snack container) no-sugar-added, natural applesauce
- ✦ 20 raw almonds
- ✦ 30 pistachios
- ✦ 2 level teaspoons natural peanut butter and a HALF fruit serving (i.e., ½ banana or 1 small apple)
- ✦ 1 level tablespoon natural peanut butter with unlimited celery sticks
- ✦ 1 slice reduced calorie, whole-grain toast (any brand, 45 calories or less per slice) with 1 level tablespoon natural peanut butter

Fruit Options

+ 1 frozen banana
+ 1 cup frozen grapes
+ One WHOLE fruit serving
+ 1 orange (or any other HALF fruit serving) and 1 mini whole-grain pita (no more than 70 calories)

Miscellaneous Options

+ 4 ounces turkey breast rolled with lettuce and mustard
+ 1 mini whole-grain pita (no more than 70 calories) with 2 level tablespoons hummus
+ ¼ cup hummus with unlimited cucumber slices, celery sticks, and/or red, yellow, and green bell pepper strips
+ 1 cup edamame beans boiled in the pod (green soybeans, fresh or frozen)

ONE PACK OF SUGARLESS GUM

I have learned from my clients that sugarless gum can be a fantastic diet tool. It prevents you from endless rounds of tasting while preparing meals, it gives your mouth something other than nibbling at cookies to do when you're bored, and it sends a blast of flavor to your taste buds. Plus—as just about everyone knows—four out of five dentists (at least!) recommend chewing sugarless gum after eating if you can't brush because it helps clear the little bits of food that get trapped between teeth. I always carry a pack in my handbag. It's a healthy "vice."

Unlimited Food/Beverage List

Enjoy in unlimited amounts—at any time of the day.

- **ALL non-starchy vegetables! (see vegetables list on pages 29–31)**
- Club soda (with optional fresh lemon or lime)
- Coffee (black, or with skim, 1%, or soy milk only; no natural or artificial sweeteners)
- Naturally flavored zero-calorie coffee with no natural or artificial sweeteners (see recipes on page 37)

SUMMER MINT TEA

Just because a beverage doesn't contain sugar, it doesn't have to be boring. For proof, try my special iced tea recipe:

4 mint tea bags
2 black tea bags
Pinch baking soda
4 cups water, boiling
4 cups water, cold
Lemon wedges (optional)

Place the tea bags and baking soda in a 2-quart pitcher. (The baking soda makes for a smoother, less bitter glass of iced tea.) Add the boiling water. Steep the tea bags for 5 to 10 minutes, depending on desired strength. Remove the tea bags and add the cold water. Cool at room temperature for at least 30 minutes before refrigerating to prevent tea from becoming cloudy. Serve over ice; garnish with lemon wedges.

- ✦ Extracts (vanilla, almond, peppermint, etc.)
- ✦ Herbs & spices (see list on pages 35–36)
- ✦ Horseradish
- ✦ Hot sauce
- ✦ Lemon and lime wedges
- ✦ Low-sodium broth
- ✦ Mustard (plain, brown, spicy, Dijon)
- ✦ Nonstick cooking spray
- ✦ Joy's *LIFE* Balsamic Vinaigrette Salad Dressing
- ✦ Salt substitute
- ✦ Seltzer water (plain or naturally flavored with optional fresh lemon or lime)
- ✦ Sparkling water
- ✦ Tea (iced or hot, with lemon or skim, 1%, or soy milk only; no natural or artificial sweeteners)
- ✦ Vinegar (any variety)
- ✦ Wasabi
- ✦ Water (with optional fresh lemon or lime)
- ✦ Naturally flavored waters, zero calorie (see recipe on page 38)

LISA DREHER

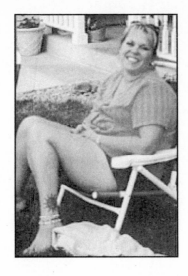 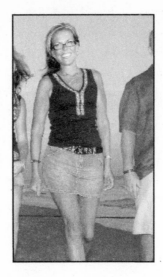

LOST: **125 pounds!**

AGE: **34**

HEIGHT: **5'7"**

BEFORE: **250 pounds, size 22**

AFTER: **125 pounds, size 4**

THIN ACCOMPLISHMENTS: Went from no exercise at all to walking seven miles and jumping rope 900 times each day.

THIN CHALLENGES: Keeping active during snowy winters.

WORDS OF WISDOM: Once it's in your head and your heart to lose weight, you can do it! And once you change the way you live your life, those new habits become as automatic as waking up and brushing your teeth or hair. It doesn't have to be a struggle for the rest of your life.

I held my father's hand while he had a heart attack. My dad is a big guy, the rock of the family. He's my best friend, and it crushed me. I went to every doctor's appointment he had, learned about what he should be doing to have a stronger heart, and decided to change my cooking style to match how he should be eating. Made up my own healthy recipes and cooked for him. My dad didn't lose his weight, but I lost mine!

WEIGHT LOSS "SECRETS"

There's no miracle involved. You have to change your entire life. When I was younger, I learned Southern cooking from my Kentucky grandmother—everything deep-fried or slathered in butter. I could go through four sticks of butter a day! No more. No butter, no sugar. My dad's doctor said that eating late at night makes the heart work harder, so I never eat after dinner. Our neighbors know that if they want to see the Drehers for a food event, they have to plan an early evening. It's a small sacrifice for my health.

THE BEST PART . . .

I feel twenty years younger, which means I get to be a teenager all over again!

JOY'S LESSONS LEARNED

Skip your late night snack. For many people, evening tends to be the time of day they go on calorie overload—comfort food central: ice cream, cookies, potato chips, popcorn, and more! Skip your nighttime snack altogether. Sip an herbal tea or chew some sugarless gum, floss or brush your teeth, and close down the kitchen for the evening.

HOW TO STICK WITH APPROPRIATE SERVING SIZES

- While you learn to eyeball appropriate portion sizes, consider investing in a small kitchen food scale. That way, you can accurately weigh out food amounts.
- For meat and poultry, ask your butcher to do some of the work. For example, request one pound of chicken breast wrapped in four 4-ounce packages and you'll have equal portions measured out for you to use immediately or to freeze.
- Whip out your measuring cups and spoons for cereal, salad dressings, condiments, cottage cheese, and yogurts.
- Buy a bunch of 1-cup and 2-cup containers. Then, use them to pre-measure your favorite items. For example, fill a 1-cup container halfway and you'll have an easy half cup of cottage cheese or rice, etc.
- Visualize appropriate amounts by comparisons to common objects. For example:

FOR PROTEIN:
- 3 ounces beef, poultry, pork or thick fish = deck of cards or palm of hand
- 3 ounces thin fish fillet = checkbook
- 5 ounces beef, poultry, pork or thick fish = approximately 1½ decks of cards

FOR DAIRY:
- ½ cup cottage cheese = half baseball or half tennis ball
- One cup cottage cheese or nonfat yogurt = one baseball or tennis ball
- One ounce reduced-fat cheese = 4 dice or your thumb

(Continued)

FOR STARCH:

- ½ cup cooked pasta or rice=small computer mouse or half baseball

FOR FAT:

- 1 teaspoon peanut butter or mayo or salad dressing=one die or tip of your thumb

Step One
Menus and Recipes

On the following pages are meal plans for the full 7 days of Step One.

Although I have planned these menus for variety and nutrition, I understand that you may not enjoy all the foods I use. Feel free to repeat or swap corresponding meals—breakfast for breakfast, lunch for lunch, or dinner for dinner (from among Step One meals *only*). If you're a member of the online program at www .JoyBauer.com, you'll be able to browse even more Step One meals and recipes.

For a list of the easiest, low-prep meals for Step One, see page 55.

In the event that you must eat out during this week, follow my LIFE Diet Step One Restaurant Options on page 56.

Special Instructions for All Men and Some Active Women

(Follow these instructions if you are a man, or if you are a woman under age 40 who does more than one hour of cardiovascular exercise at least six days each week.) Although specific portions are listed for protein at each meal (egg whites, meat, chicken, turkey, fish and seafood, tofu), all men and active women may eat *unlimited* protein portions at meals only—that means breakfast, lunch, and dinner, but not with your snack or throughout the rest of the day.

Special Instructions for Vegetarians

Substitute low-fat soy milk, soy yogurt, and soy cheese for dairy products. For meat and poultry, substitute an equivalent portion of fish, seafood, tempeh, or meat analog products. If opting to replace meat with tofu, double the portion size listed (since tofu is less dense than meat). You may also substitute veggie burgers for turkey burgers or other meat entrées.

BREAKFAST

Egg-cellent Omelet with Vegetables & Cheese (page 57)

~ and ~

one WHOLE serving your choice of approved fruit

LUNCH

California-Style Turkey Sandwich

1 slice whole grain bread or 2 slices reduced calorie whole wheat bread (any brand 45 calories or less per slice); 4 ounces turkey breast; 2 thin slices avocado; unlimited tomato slices, lettuce, arugula, and/or spinach; mustard

Baby Carrots

unlimited

SNACK

Cottage cheese and bell pepper strips

½ cup nonfat or 1% low-fat cottage cheese

unlimited sliced green, red, and/or yellow bell pepper strips

DINNER

LIFE Dinner Salad (page 59)

~ or ~

2 cups *LIFE* Veggie Soup (page 63)

Grilled Fish with Salsa

6 ounces baked or grilled white fish (halibut, cod, or tilapia); ¼ cup mild or spicy salsa

Green vegetable

Unlimited steamed asparagus spears, broccoli, sugar snap peas, or green beans

HALF serving of any approved fruit

(¾ cup fresh berries, 1 cup cubed melon, ½ cup frozen grapes, or 1 orange)

BREAKFAST

Cereal with Milk

1 cup whole grain cereal (any brand 150 calories or less per 1 cup serving and 3+grams fiber); 1 cup skim milk or low-fat soy milk

HALF serving of any approved fruit

(tasty options include 1 orange, ½ grapefruit, ½ banana, or 2 tablespoons raisins)

LUNCH

Chicken Caesar Salad

Unlimited Romaine lettuce (chopped); 4 ounces grilled skinless chicken breast; 3 tablespoons grated Parmesan cheese; 4 tablespoons light Caesar dressing (any brand 80 calories or less per 2 tablespoons)

SNACK

1 ounce reduced-fat or nonfat cheese and 1 rice cake

DINNER

LIFE Dinner Salad (page 59)

~ or ~

2 cups *LIFE* Veggie Soup (page 63)

Grilled Sirloin Steak

5 ounces lean sirloin steak, seasoned as desired with allowed marinades/herbs/seasonings.

Pre-heat a large skillet or grill to medium-high heat and cook to preferred temperature.

Sautéed Spinach (page 65)

BREAKFAST
Vanilla Pumpkin Pudding (page 57)

LUNCH
Turkey Burger on Greens

>5-ounce* turkey burger served on a bed of mixed greens or spinach
(unlimited amounts) with lettuce, tomato, onion, and/or pickle

>2 tablespoons ketchup or salsa (optional)

>* enjoy any standard turkey burger or use E-Z Turkey Burger recipe on page 68

Raw or steamed vegetables

>Your choice unlimited amounts approved veggies

SNACK

>1 small apple + 10 raw almonds or 15 pistachios

DINNER
LIFE Dinner Salad (page 59)
~ or ~
2 cups *LIFE* Veggie Soup (pages 63–64)
Your Choice Teriyaki of
Beef, Salmon, Chicken, *or* Tofu (pages 65–67)

BREAKFAST
PB-Fruit Toast
2 slices reduced-calorie whole wheat toast with 2 level teaspoons peanut, almond, or soy nut butter spread (1 teaspoon for each slice) topped with one HALF serving of any approved fruit of your choice (tasty options: ½ sliced banana or ¾ cup blueberries, raspberries, or sliced strawberries)

LUNCH
Broccoli & Cheese Omelet (page 59)
Mixed Green Salad
Unlimited lettuce and/or spinach leaves with
2 tablespoons light dressing (40 calories or less per 2 tablespoons)
~ or ~
*2 tablespoons of any of Joy's **LIFE** dressings (pages 60–63)*
~ or ~
1 teaspoon olive oil with unlimited vinegar or fresh lemon

SNACK
1 cup fresh or frozen edamame (green soybeans) boiled in the pod

DINNER
LIFE Dinner Salad (page 59)
~ or ~
2 cups *LIFE* Veggie Soup (page 63)
Pork Tenderloin with Steamed Veggies
5 ounces grilled, roasted, or broiled lean pork tenderloin, seasoned as desired with unlimited steamed asparagus spears, snow peas or green string beans

HALF serving of any fruit of your choice
(tasty options include ½ grapefruit, 1 orange, 1 small apple, 1 peach, or 1 nectarine)

BREAKFAST

Cottage Cheese with Berries

1 cup nonfat or 1% low-fat cottage cheese topped with 2 tablespoons wheat germ and mixed with a HALF serving of fruit (tasty options include ¾ cup berries, ½ cup fresh pineapple, 1 small apple, or ½ banana)

LUNCH

Tuna Salad with Pita (page 58)

~ and ~

Side veggies

Unlimited cucumber slices, pepper strips, and celery sticks

SNACK

30 pistachio nuts or 20 raw almonds

DINNER

LIFE Dinner Salad (page 59)

~ or ~

2 cups *LIFE* Veggie Soup (page 63)

Grilled Chicken Parmesan (page 69)

~ and ~

Steamed Broccoli

unlimited

BREAKFAST

Oatmeal with Fruit

> ½ cup dry traditional oatmeal (or ¼ cup steel cut oats) prepared with water
>
> Top with a HALF serving of any fruit of your choice
>
> (tasty options include ¾ cup fresh berries or 1 small apple, chopped)

~ and ~

2 large hardboiled egg whites (discard yolks)

LUNCH

Open-Faced Toasted Tomato and Cheese Sandwich

> 2 slices reduced-calorie whole wheat bread (any brand 45 calories or less per slice), toasted and each topped with sliced tomato and 1 slice (¾ to 1 ounce) reduced-fat cheese
>
> Place in the oven or under the broiler until the cheese melts.

Baby Carrots

SNACK

Naked Turkey Roll-up

> Lay down unlimited large leaves of lettuce (such as Romaine).
>
> Top with 4 ounces turkey breast and mustard, roll and eat with your fingers.

DINNER

LIFE Dinner Salad (page 59)

~ or ~

2 cups *LIFE* Veggie Soup (page 63)

Grilled Salmon

> 5 ounces wild salmon fillet grilled with 1 teaspoon olive oil, fresh lemon, and choice of approved seasonings

Cauliflower Mash (page 69)

> 1 serving (¾ cup)
>
> (can substitute unlimited steamed cauliflower, broccoli, or Brussels sprouts)

BREAKFAST
Skinny Burrito Pocket (page 58)

LUNCH
Cottage Cheese and Fruit Combo

> 1 cup nonfat or 1% low-fat cottage cheese with 2 tablespoons wheat germ
>
> Enjoy with one WHOLE serving of your choice of fruit
>
> (tasty options include ½ medium cantaloupe, 1 large apple, 1½ cups berries, ½ large mango sliced, or 1 banana)

SNACK

> 1 level tablespoon natural peanut butter + unlimited celery sticks

DINNER
LIFE Dinner Salad (page 59)

~ or ~

2 cups LIFE Veggie Soup (page 63)
Cheddar Turkey Burger with Sautéed Mushrooms (page 68)

BREAKFASTS

Cereal with Milk and Fruit (Day 2)

Vanilla Pumpkin Pudding (Day 3)

PB-Fruit Toast (Day 4)

LUNCHES

California-Style Turkey Sandwich (Day 1)

Bonus Timesaver: Leave off the avocado and add a slice of reduced-fat cheese.

Tuna Salad with Pita (Day 5)

Bonus Timesaver: For your side veggies, use baby carrots straight from the bag.

Open Faced Toasted Tomato and Cheese Sandwich (Day 6)

Bonus Timesaver: Microwave this sandwich instead of broiling if you're making it away from home. Or, simply enjoy it cold.

DINNERS

LIFE Salad (every day)

Bonus Timesaver: Open a pre-washed bag of salad and drizzle on low-cal dressing or plain balsamic vinegar.

Grilled Sirloin Steak with Sautéed Spinach (Day 2)

Bonus Timesaver: Microwave a box of frozen chopped spinach in place of sautéed spinach.

Grilled Chicken Parmesan with Steamed Broccoli (Day 5)

Cheddar Turkey Burger with Sautéed Mushrooms (Day 7)

Bonus Timesaver: Purchase frozen turkey burgers or fresh ground turkey already formed into patties and skip the sautéed mushrooms.

easiest meals at-a-glance

Joy's LIFE Diet Step One Restaurant Options

Some Step One menu options can easily be ordered in a restaurant, as long as you are willing to make a few special requests about how the foods are prepared. But there are also some generic meals you can order anytime and nearly anywhere. (Always remember: If it is not listed here or in the Unlimited Foods list, don't eat it! For example, don't eat bread, rice, extra fruit, full-fat salad dressings, sauces, etc.)

Breakfast

Egg white omelet stuffed with any of your favorite vegetables (no cheese—most restaurants don't offer reduced-fat cheese), *plus* ½ grapefruit or ¼ cantaloupe, or side portion of fresh berries or fruit salad.

Coffee (black, or with skim or 1% milk only) or tea (iced or hot, unsweetened, with lemon *or* skim or 1% milk only).

Lunch

Large salad piled with raw vegetables and topped with skinless grilled chicken *or* turkey *or* shrimp (no cheese). Use plain balsamic or red wine vinegar *or* fresh lemon (with optional 1 teaspoon olive oil—that's two dashes from a bottle) as dressing, or 2 tablespoons low-calorie dressing (if available).

Water, seltzer, coffee (black, or with skim or 1% milk only), and/or tea (iced or hot, unsweetened, with lemon *or* skim or 1% milk only).

Dinner

House salad with plain vinegar or fresh lemon.

Skinless chicken breast *or* fish *or* seafood *or* pork tenderloin *or* turkey *or* lean steak (all options must be grilled, baked, roasted, poached, steamed, or boiled *only*).

Double order of steamed, plain non-starchy vegetables.

Water, seltzer, tea (iced or hot, unsweetened, with lemon *or* skim or 1% milk only). Great after-dinner choices include all herbal teas (especially mint or chamomile) and green tea.

EGG-CELLENT OMELET WITH VEGETABLES & CHEESE

Any amount diced veggies—any from approved list. Popular choices include
   onion, bell pepper, tomato, mushrooms, broccoli, and spinach
3 large egg whites
Your choice approved seasonings
¼ cup (1 ounce) shredded reduced-fat or nonfat cheese

In a pan sprayed with nonstick cooking spray, sauté the veggies over medium heat until tender.

Whip the egg whites and pour over the sautéed vegetables.

Add preferred seasonings and continue to cook. When the bottom side is cooked, gently flip and cook the other side.

Add the cheese and fold one side over the other.

Makes one serving

VANILLA PUMPKIN PUDDING

8 ounces nonfat vanilla yogurt
½ cup canned 100% pure pumpkin puree (no added sugar)
1 tablespoon slivered almonds or chopped walnuts
Dash cinnamon

In a small bowl, blend or layer the yogurt and pumpkin.

Top with nuts and cinnamon.

Makes one serving

SKINNY BURRITO POCKET

½ cup diced peppers and/or onions

1 teaspoon minced jalapeno (optional)

3 egg whites

¼ cup black beans, rinsed well

2 tablespoons shredded reduced-fat or fat-free cheese

1 small whole grain pita (any brand 70 calories or less)

Salsa or hot sauce (optional)

In pan sprayed with nonstick cooking spray, sauté the peppers and onions over medium heat until tender.

Whip the egg whites, add to the pan, and scramble.

Remove the cooked eggs from the heat and mix with black beans and cheese.

Slice the closed pita in half, and stuff each half with half the egg mixture.

Add the salsa or hot sauce.

Makes one serving

Recipes—Lunch and Snacks

TUNA SALAD WITH PITA

1 mini whole wheat pita (any brand 70 calories or less per pita)

1 6-ounce can water-packed light tuna

3 tablespoons nonfat Greek yogurt or 1 tablespoon reduced-fat mayo

¼ teaspoon dried dill weed or other desired seasonings

Lettuce, tomato, radish, and/or cucumber

Squeeze of fresh lemon (optional)

Split pita in half and toast lightly.

Mix the tuna, yogurt or mayo, and seasoning. Top the pita with the tuna mixture, open-face style, and add the lettuce, tomato, radish, and cucumber. Squeeze the lemon on top.

Enjoy with unlimited amounts of cucumber slices, pepper strips, and celery sticks on the side.

Makes one serving

BROCCOLI & CHEESE OMELET

1 cup broccoli florets

4 egg whites

Your choice approved seasonings

¼ cup (1 oz) shredded reduced-fat or nonfat cheese

In a pan sprayed with nonstick cooking spray, sauté the broccoli over medium heat until tender.

Whip the egg whites and pour over the sautéed broccoli.

Add preferred seasonings and continue to cook. When bottom side is cooked, gently flip and cook the other side.

Add the cheese and fold one side over the other.

Makes one serving

Recipes—Dinner and Sides

Every dinner in Step One should begin with your choice of either the Step One Dinner Salad or 2 cups of *LIFE* Veggie Soup. These meal starters are designed to add plenty of volume and fiber to your meal and keep you from overindulging at dinner or later in the evening, so don't skip this important element.

LIFE DINNER SALAD

Start with a bed of Romaine lettuce, spinach, or mixed greens.

Add your preferred blend of non-starchy vegetables. Choose from:
- Carrots
- Celery

- ✦ Tomatoes
- ✦ Onions
- ✦ Radishes
- ✦ Mushrooms
- ✦ Cucumbers
- ✦ Bell peppers
- ✦ Your choice—use whatever nonstarchy veggies you already have on hand in your fridge. *If you're following the plan, you should have loads of options—half a tomato left over from lunch, a small handful of baby carrots, etc. Just add whatever's convenient that night.*

For dressing, choose one of the following:

- ✦ 2 tablespoons light dressing (any brand 40 calories or less per 2 tablespoons)
- ✦ 1 teaspoon olive oil, with unlimited balsamic vinegar, red wine vinegar, or fresh lemon
- ✦ 2 tablespoons of any of Joy's *LIFE* dressings
- ✦ Unlimited amounts of plain vinegar (red wine or balsamic) or fresh lemon or Joy's *LIFE* Balsamic Vinaigrette dressing.

Joy's LIFE Dressings

BALSAMIC VINAIGRETTE

1 clove garlic, minced (1 teaspoon), or ¼ teaspoon garlic powder

2 tablespoons Dijon mustard

2 tablespoons balsamic vinegar

1 tablespoon fresh lemon juice

1 tablespoon water

Combine all the ingredients in a small bowl and whisk them together well. Keep refrigerated in airtight container for up to 1 week.

Makes approximately 3 servings, 2 tablespoons each

RASPBERRY VINAIGRETTE

2 tablespoons raspberry jam, all fruit

2 tablespoons Dijon mustard

2 tablespoons balsamic vinegar

4 tablespoons water

Combine all the ingredients in a small bowl and whisk them together well. The vinaigrette will keep for up to 1 week if refrigerated in an airtight container.

Makes approximately 5 servings, 2 tablespoons each

THOUSAND ISLAND DRESSING

3 tablespoons reduced-fat mayo (any brand 25 calories or less per tablespoon)

2 tablespoons ketchup

½ teaspoon Worcestershire sauce

1 tablespoon pickle relish

½ teaspoon horseradish (optional)

Combine all the ingredients in a small bowl and whisk together well. The dressing will keep for up to 1 week if refrigerated in an airtight container.

Makes approximately 3 servings, 2 tablespoons each

CAESAR DRESSING

¾ cup low-fat buttermilk

1 clove garlic, minced (or 1 teaspoon), or ¼ teaspoon garlic powder

½ cup grated Parmesan cheese

1 anchovy fillet (optional)

2 tablespoons cider vinegar

1 teaspoon coarsely ground black pepper

Add all the ingredients to a blender and puree until smooth. Refrigerate for 30 minutes before serving. The dressing will keep for up to 1 week if refrigerated in an airtight container.

Makes approximately 9 servings, 2 tablespoons each

TOMATO PARMESAN DRESSING

½ cup tomato or vegetable juice (no salt added)

1 clove garlic, minced (1 teaspoon), or ¼ teaspoon garlic powder

2 teaspoons grated Parmesan cheese

1 teaspoon finely chopped sun-dried tomato (oil-packed)

½ teaspoon red wine vinegar

⅛ teaspoon dried basil leaves

⅛ teaspoon dried oregano leaves

¼ teaspoon salt

Pinch dried thyme

Black pepper

Combine all the ingredients in a small bowl and whisk them together well. The dressing will keep for up to 1 week if refrigerated in an airtight container.

Makes approximately 5 servings, 2 tablespoons each

ORANGE GINGER DRESSING

¼ cup orange juice

½ teaspoon grated fresh ginger root

1 clove garlic, minced (1 teaspoon), or ¼ teaspoon garlic powder

2 tablespoons hoisin sauce

1 teaspoon rice wine vinegar

¼ teaspoon sesame seeds

⅛ teaspoon orange zest, grated (optional)

Combine all the ingredients in a small bowl and whisk them together well. The dressing will keep for up to 1 week if refrigerated in an airtight container.

Makes approximately 3 servings, 2 tablespoons each

CREAMY GARLIC DILL DRESSING

½ cup low-fat buttermilk

2 tablespoons fat-free sour cream

2 teaspoons white wine vinegar

1 clove garlic, minced (1 teaspoon), or ¼ teaspoon garlic powder

1 tablespoon chopped fresh dill or 1 teaspoon dried dill

¼ teaspoon salt

Ground pepper (preferably white pepper)

Combine all the ingredients in a small bowl and whisk them together well. The dressing will keep for up to 1 week if refrigerated in an airtight container.

Makes approximately 6 servings, 2 tablespoons each

MAPLE DIJON DRESSING

1 clove garlic, minced (1 teaspoon), or ¼ teaspoon garlic powder

2 tablespoons Dijon mustard

2 tablespoons real maple syrup

1 tablespoon cider vinegar

½ lime, juiced (about 1 tablespoon)

Combine all the ingredients in a small bowl and whisk them together well. The dressing will keep for up to 1 week if refrigerated in an airtight container.

Makes approximately 3 servings, 2 tablespoons each

LIFE VEGGIE SOUP

Enjoy in place of the *LIFE* Dinner Salad any night of the week. Feel free to omit any vegetables you don't enjoy and replace with other non-starchy vegetables (see list of allowed vegetables, pages 29–31). Prepare this soup at the beginning of Step One and divide into 2-cup portions. You can store individual portions in the fridge for up to 3 days (any longer and the veggies will become too soggy) or freeze for up to 1 month and defrost as needed.

4 cloves garlic, minced (4 teaspoons)

1 onion, diced (1 cup)

3 celery stalks, diced (1½ cups)

1 package (8 ounces) sliced mushrooms

8 cups (2 quarts) low-sodium chicken or vegetable stock

1 cup sliced carrots (frozen or fresh)

1 zucchini, diced (2 cups)

1 cup chopped green beans, fresh or frozen

2 cups chopped cauliflower florets, fresh or frozen (½ medium head)

3 cups cabbage, roughly chopped (½ cabbage head)

1 can diced tomato (15 oz), preferably no salt added

3 bay leaves

2 tablespoons red wine vinegar (or balsamic vinegar)

Choose one seasoning blend:

> *Creole: 2 teaspoons basil, 1 teaspoon oregano, 1 tablespoon paprika, 1 teaspoon black pepper, ¼ teaspoon cayenne pepper, ½ teaspoon thyme*
>
> *Italian: 2 teaspoons dried parsley, 2 teaspoons basil, 1 teaspoon oregano, ½ teaspoon thyme, ½ teaspoon sage, ½ teaspoon black pepper*
>
> *Garden Herbs: 2 tablespoons chopped thyme, ¼ cup freshly chopped parsley, ¼ cup freshly chopped basil*

1. In a large, nonstick stock pot coated with cooking spray, sauté the garlic, onion, celery, and mushrooms over medium heat for 10 minutes, or until tender.

2. Add the stock, carrots, zucchini, green beans, cauliflower florets, cabbage, canned tomatoes, and bay leaves. If you have chosen one of the dry seasoning blends (Creole or Italian) add it now. Bring to a boil, cover, and simmer over low heat for 20 minutes.

3. Add the vinegar and cook for an additional 2 minutes. If you have chosen the Garden Herbs seasoning blend, add it now. Remove the bay leaves before serving or freezing.

4. Storage/Freezing Directions: Allow soup to cool to room temperature. This recipe can be prepared up to 3 days in advance and stored in the fridge. Two-cup portions may be frozen and stored for up to a month.

Recipe yields 12 cups, or six 2-cup portions.

SAUTÉED SPINACH

1 teaspoon olive oil

1 clove garlic, diced (optional)

4 cups spinach leaves

Your choice approved seasonings

Coat a pan with nonstick cooking spray. Add the olive oil, and heat to medium. Add the garlic.

Add the spinach leaves and sauté until cooked down.

Season as desired with approved seasonings.

Makes one serving

BEEF TERIYAKI

1 clove garlic, minced (1 teaspoon) or ¼ teaspoon garlic powder

1 teaspoon finely minced or grated fresh ginger root; or ⅛ teaspoon ground ginger

2 tablespoons low-sodium teriyaki sauce

¼ teaspoon red pepper flakes

½ teaspoon ground coriander seed

5 ounce lean sirloin steak, cut across grain in thin slices

½ cup Savoy cabbage, thinly sliced

½ cup red bell pepper cut in thin strips

½ cup fresh bean sprouts

Combine the garlic, ginger, teriyaki sauce, red pepper, and coriander in a small flat dish.

Add the sirloin and cover it thoroughly with marinade. Refrigerate for 10 to 20 minutes. (For a deeper flavor, marinate for 3 hours or overnight.)

Coat a medium fry pan with cooking spray, place on moderate heat. Add the sirloin slices. Cook to desired doneness.

Add the cabbage and bell pepper and combine well with the beef and marinade. Cover the pan and cook for 5 to 7 minutes. Add the bean sprouts and cook for another 3 minutes.

Makes one serving

SALMON TERIYAKI

2 tablespoons low-sodium teriyaki sauce

1 teaspoon finely minced or grated fresh ginger root or ⅛ teaspoon ground ginger

Black pepper

5 ounce salmon fillet

1 cup snow peas

1 tablespoon finely chopped fresh chives (optional)

Combine the teriyaki sauce, ginger, and black pepper in a small flat dish.

Add the salmon fillet to the dish and cover with marinade on both sides. Refrigerate for 10 to 20 minutes.

Preheat the oven to 400°F. Heat a small sauté pan coated with nonstick spray over medium high heat.

Place the salmon fillet in fry pan, skin side up. Allow to cook until browned, about 3 minutes. Turn over and cook for an additional 2 to 3 minutes. If fry pan is oven-proof, place directly in preheated oven. If not, place salmon in small oven-proof dish before placing in oven. Bake for 7 to 10 minutes, or until flesh is opaque and salmon is fully cooked.

While salmon is in oven, steam snow peas over boiling water for 7 to 8 minutes. Transfer snow peas and salmon to plate and garnish with chopped chives.

Makes one serving

CHICKEN TERIYAKI

6 ounces boneless skinless chicken breast, cut into thin strips

3 tablespoons low-sodium teriyaki sauce

1 clove garlic, minced (1 teaspoon); or ¼ teaspoon garlic powder

1 teaspoon fresh ginger root, finely minced or grated; or ⅛ teaspoon ground ginger

Black pepper

½ cup red bell pepper, cut into thin strips

½ cup snow peas, cut into thin strips

1 cup broccoli, cut into small, equal sized pieces

Combine teriyaki sauce, garlic, ginger, and black pepper in small bowl.

Add chicken strips to bowl and combine thoroughly with marinade. Refrigerate for at least 30 minutes or overnight.

Heat small sauté pan coated with nonstick spray over medium heat. Add chicken and marinade to pan and cook thoroughly, until chicken is no longer pink. Add vegetables, cover pan, and cook for approximately 7 minutes.

Makes one serving

TOFU TERIYAKI

1 tablespoon plus 1 tablespoon low-sodium teriyaki sauce

1 clove garlic, minced (1 teaspoon), or ¼ teaspoon garlic powder

1 teaspoon fresh ginger root, finely minced or grated; or ⅛ teaspoon ground ginger

Black pepper

6 ounces firm tofu—cut into ¼" slices

1 cup snow peas, cut into thin strips

½ cup red bell pepper, cut into thin strips

1 cup thinly sliced Savoy cabbage

1 cup broccoli, cut into small equal sized pieces

Combine 1 tablespoon of teriyaki sauce, garlic, ginger, and black pepper in small bowl.

Add the tofu slices to the bowl and combine thoroughly with marinade. Refrigerate for 20 to 30 minutes.

Heat a small sauté pan coated with nonstick spray over medium heat. Add the tofu slices and the marinade to the pan and brown the tofu on both sides.

Add the snow peas, bell pepper, cabbage, broccoli, and remaining 1 tablespoon of teriyaki sauce to the pan. Cover and cook for 5 to 7 minutes.

Makes one serving

E-Z TURKEY BURGER

1 pound lean ground turkey (at least 90% lean)

¼ cup ketchup (4 tablespoons)

1 tablespoon Dijon or spicy brown mustard

1 teaspoon garlic powder

1 chopped onion (optional)

Combine all the ingredients. Divide the mixture into 4 equal-sized portions and shape into burgers.

Grill or broil the turkey burgers until cooked through, about 5 to 7 minutes on each side. Serve without bun.

Makes 4 burgers

CHEDDAR TURKEY BURGER WITH SAUTÉED MUSHROOMS

1 cup sliced mushrooms (Portobello, Baby Bella/Crimini, or white button mushrooms)

5 ounce turkey burger

1 ounce reduced-fat or nonfat cheddar cheese, sliced (if desired, substitute Swiss for cheddar)

Lettuce, tomato, onion, pickle (all optional)

Thoroughly coat a small sauté pan with nonstick cooking spray.

Add the mushrooms and sauté over medium heat until soft, about 5 minutes. Set aside.

Grill or broil the turkey burger until cooked through, about 5 to 7 minutes on each side. Top with cheese, mushrooms, lettuce, tomato, onion, and pickle. Skip the bun!

Makes one serving

CAULIFLOWER MASHED "POTATOES"

1 large head cauliflower, cut into florets of roughly the same size

2 tablespoons fat-free cream cheese

2 tablespoons grated Romano or Parmesan cheese

¼ teaspoon garlic powder

Pinch nutmeg

Ground black pepper

Salt substitute (optional)

Steam the cauliflower over boiling water for 10 to 15 minutes, until tender. Or microwave on high for 10 to 15 minutes or until very tender. Drain thoroughly.

For lumpy consistency: Mash with a fork and thoroughly blend in the cream cheese, grated cheese, garlic powder, and nutmeg. Season with black pepper and salt substitute to taste.

For creamier consistency: Place the cauliflower in a food processor with the cream cheese, grated cheese, garlic powder, and nutmeg. Puree on high until smooth. Season with black pepper and salt substitute.

Makes 4 servings, ¾ cup each

GRILLED CHICKEN PARMESAN

5 ounce chicken breast

2 tablespoons marinara sauce

1 ounce part-skim shredded mozzarella cheese

Grill or sauté the chicken breast in a pan sprayed with nonstick cooking spray over medium heat until cooked through.

Top the cooked chicken breast with marinara sauce and cheese, and broil until hot and bubbly (or microwave for 30 seconds to melt cheese).

Makes one serving

PAM & DAVID GROSSE

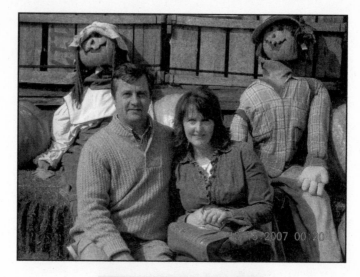

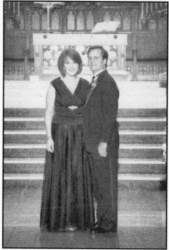

PAM GROSSE	DAVID GROSSE
LOST: **14 pounds!**	LOST: **23 pounds!**
AGE: **51**	AGE: **52**
HEIGHT: **5'5"**	HEIGHT: **5'9"**
BEFORE: **151 pounds**	BEFORE: **192 pounds**
AFTER: **137 pounds**	AFTER: **169 pounds**

THIN ACCOMPLISHMENTS: Lost weight in time for our daughter's wedding.

THIN CHALLENGES: Overcoming fifty years (each!) of generally bad eating habits.

FINALLY GETTING STARTED: We always said we would diet "tomorrow," but tomorrow never actually arrived. The wedding gave us a deadline we could shoot for. We both worked with Joy Bauer to take off 20 pounds each before our daughter's wedding. We began Joy's diet on January 1, and reported our progress just after the early May wedding.

DID YOU MEET YOUR GOALS OF 20 POUNDS EACH?

DAVID: I did!

PAM: No, I only lost 14 pounds, but that was my choice. I actually chose to taper off because I was worried that I would have to have my dress altered before the wedding. I didn't want to try it on a week before and discover that it was too big. The dress fit beautifully, and I didn't want to worry about that detail. Now that the wedding is over, I've started again and I know I'll make my goal.

WHAT MADE YOU DECIDE TO TRY THIS DIET?

PAM: I'd put on 12 pounds after my hysterectomy, and I have had a hard time getting my body regulated. I noticed that David's stomach was sticking out a bit. Heart disease runs in his family, so it was kind of scaring me.

DAVID: I had a gut. I picked shirts I didn't have to tuck in. When I looked in the mirror, I kept looking for a good angle. I never had a weight problem when I was younger, so I never understood it. I just didn't have the drive until Pam went on Joy's diet—and told me that I was going to be going on it with her.

WAS IT DIFFICULT?

DAVID: It took me about three weeks to get used to eating different food. I had a personal commitment, though, and I was going to get this thing done.

PAM: It was more about eliminating bad habits. I have a real sweet tooth. I used to eat a handful of M&Ms and feel like I hadn't eaten anything, but the calories add up . . . and up. It was difficult for me not to snack all day long.

DAVID: I learned about portion control. I used to eat a huge plate of food and then go back for seconds. It wasn't fun adjusting to smaller portions, but you know what the reward is? When you can take your pants to the tailor and they cut two inches off the waist. I used to think I didn't want to be controlled by a diet, but you know what? With my old way of eating, the food was controlling me. It controlled the way I felt about myself. I feel much better now.

PAM: I had the mindset that maybe I was too old to take the weight off, and that maybe weight didn't matter at my age anymore. I was not in a good mood in the early part of the diet. I dreaded meals. I wished we could just go out and eat fried chicken. I'm not sure I would have kept going if David wasn't doing it with me. But once I started losing weight, that certainly kept me motivated. I said, "If I can't do it for this wedding, I'll never do it."

DO YOU MISS YOUR OLD WAY OF EATING?

PAM: I used to say I could live on sugar. Now I look at things like that and say, it's not worth it. I'd rather be healthy, and I've learned to love healthier treats.

DAVID: It took a couple of months before I could honestly say this, but those old unhealthy habits are gone for good. This is a new lifestyle for us.

JOY'S LESSONS LEARNED

RECRUIT YOUR SIGNIFICANT OTHER AND LOSE WEIGHT TOGETHER.
Studies show that negative habits, like gaining weight, are contagious. Pam and David prove that positive habits are contagious as well. So go out and recruit a weight loss partner.

Step Two—*Relearn*

2

hey say that once you learn to ride a bike, you never forget. Even decades later, the minute your feet hit the pedals your body will go into automatic pilot mode and you'll be flying down the street like you were born to ride. This wondrous combination of muscle memory and habit persists long after we outgrow that first two-wheeler, almost as if it had been physically carved into some little corner of our brains.

We depend on this hardwiring of habit to get through our days. Life would be incredibly burdensome if we had to concentrate on how to brush our teeth, open a door, turn on a light switch, sign our name, et cetera, et cetera. Eating fits into that list, too. Our food habits are etched into our bodies and brains from very early in our lives. This memory includes everything—which hand holds the fork, how slowly you chew, food preparation methods, portion judgment, and taste preferences. And just like riding a bicycle, once we learn, we never forget. However . . . that doesn't mean you can't develop new habits and memories.

In Step One, you committed to a fresh start by recognizing and releasing negative food habits. Step Two involves *relearning*, laying down a new set of patterns for making food choices for weight loss, eating healthier portions, and exploring some fresh tastes. It's the next phase in a progression. You learned to ride a tricycle, and then a bicycle. It's time to learn to ride a unicycle. Metaphorically, of course.

Step Two Rules

For Step Two, follow the same basic rules as Step One (you're used to them by now, right?). You can eat all the same foods, and you should feel free to repeat any of the menus and recipes you've enjoyed, but there are also some fantastic additions.

Here are additional things you'll enjoy on this phase of the plan:

1. *Expanded approved foods.* In the list below, you'll see all the approved foods, including the Step One foods, and some new ones highlighted in bold type. Continue to have no starch with dinner, and continue to start each dinner with either the *LIFE* Veggie Soup or *LIFE* Dinner Salad.

   Along with adding specific entries to your list of allowed foods, Step Two also loosens up on sweeteners, frozen dinners, and treats . . . as long as you follow the rules.

2. *Sugar substitutes and artificial sweeteners.* Moderate amounts of artificial sweetener are now allowed, but certainly not required or suggested. If you want to incorporate sweetener, Step Two allows for no more than a total of two items with artificial sweetener each day. So if you choose to drink a diet beverage, you may also have Splenda in your coffee *or* a yogurt with aspartame or sucralose. As before, all calorie-containing sweeteners are not allowed, including all sugars (white, brown, or raw) and honey, unless specifically noted in your meal plan.

3. *Prepared frozen meals.* You now have the option to eat a prepared frozen meal for dinner, as long as it contains no more than 350 calories per entrée. Try to select a dinner that is starch-free, and don't forget to eat a dinner salad or a serving of *LIFE* Veggie Soup before eating the frozen dinner!

4. *LIFE Healthy Extra.* In Step Two, you may now enjoy a preapproved treat once each day (any time you'd like). Choose from among the goodies on my approved list.

Step Two *LIFE* Healthy Extras

Healthy "fun" foods are an important part of Joy's LIFE Diet. Here in Step Two, these foods, called *LIFE* Healthy Extras, help you to *relearn* how to enjoy a wider spectrum of foods without overindulging in enjoyable treats. When choosing specific foods, read labels and choose brands that contain no more than 150 calories per serving. *LIFE* Healthy Extras include:

- One WHOLE serving of fruit, either plain or with 2 generous tablespoons reduced-fat whipped topping
- 1 medium banana, sliced, with 2 tablespoons light chocolate syrup for dipping
- 1 baked apple with 1 teaspoon sugar and cinnamon
- 1 cup natural, unsweetened applesauce
- ½ cup low-fat or fat-free pudding (any flavor or brand, or see recipes for homemade vanilla and chocolate versions on page 136)
- 6 ounces nonfat plain or Greek yogurt with 2 teaspoons honey or 1 tablespoon fruit jam
- 1 serving (20 each) savory almonds (recipe on page 133)
- 1 low-fat ice cream pop
- 1 frozen 100% fruit juice bar
- ½ cup low-fat ice cream, frozen yogurt, or sorbet
- 1 small bag soy crisps (150 calories or less)
- 1 ounce vegetable chips (150 calories or less)
- 4 cups low-fat popcorn (any prepared or microwaveable brand 30 calories or less per cup, with or without low-calorie *LIFE* seasoning blends). For homemade varieties, see recipes on page 134.
- 1 ounce dark chocolate (preferably at least 70% cocoa)
- 5 ounces red or white wine
- 5 ounces champagne
- 12 ounces light beer
- 1½ ounces vodka, gin, or tequila
- One *LIFE* Muffin (see recipes on pages 119–123)

- One *LIFE* Smoothie (see recipes on pages 132–133)
- One Joy Bauer *LIFE* Bar
- Grapefruit Rosemary Granita (recipe on page 135)
- Blueberry Mango Sorbet (recipe on page 135)
- Funky Monkey Coffee Drink (recipe on page 137)
- One low-fat hot cocoa packet mixed with 6 ounces nonfat plain or Greek yogurt (chilled or semi-frozen)
- One serving low-fat hot cocoa with any HALF fruit serving
- Chocolate covered strawberries: 1 ounce dark chocolate melted over 5 whole strawberries
- ¼ cup roasted edamame (also called roasted soybeans)
- Any afternoon snack listed on the Step Two approved snack list (pages 38–40)

Step Two Food Rules: *Dos and Don'ts*

To summarize, here are the Dos and Don'ts for Step Two. Some of these rules will look familiar because you have already been living with them for the past seven days.

✗ 1. **DON'T** . . . add sugar, honey, or other natural sweeteners to anything unless specified on the plan or in a recipe.

✗ 2. **DON'T** . . . drink alcohol unless it's your *LIFE* Healthy Extra for the day.

✗ 3. **DON'T** . . . eat any foods that are *not* on the "Allowed" list.

✗ 4. **DON'T** . . . eat starches with dinner.

✗ 5. **DON'T** . . . add salt to anything unless specified in a recipe.

✗ 6. **DON'T** . . . skip meals.

Now, the dos:

✓ 1. **DO** . . . eat on a schedule and enjoy three meals and your afternoon snack each day.

✓ 2. **DO** . . . drink lots of water throughout the day, including two 8-ounce glasses *before* lunch and two 8-ounce glasses *before* dinner. (These before-meal waters should be consumed up to 30 minutes before eating.) Enjoy as much additional water as you want during meals and throughout the day.

✓ 3. **DO** . . . begin dinner with *LIFE* Dinner Salad or *LIFE* Veggie Soup (see recipes on pages 59, 63).

✓ 4. **DO** . . . indulge in foods on the Unlimited List (pages 41–42). You can enjoy these foods in unlimited quantities at any time throughout the day, particularly when you get hungry between designated meal and snack times.

✓ 5. **DO** . . . feel free to swap meals or ingredients from within the same categories.

✓ 6. **DO** . . . enjoy meals listed in *LIFE* Restaurant Options when dining out (page 56).

✓ 7. **DO** . . . try different recipes for variety.

✓ 8. **DO** . . . feel free to repeat a favorite meal or recipe during the week, as many times as you like (including menus from Step One).

✓ 9. **DO** . . . feel free (if you choose) to consume up to two items each day with artificial sweetener or natural no-calorie sweetener.

✓ 10. **DO** . . . feel free to enjoy one *LIFE* Healthy Extra each day at any time you like.

✓ 11. **DO** . . . feel free to substitute a frozen entrée for dinner on any night, as long as it's 350 calories or less. No-starch entrées are strongly recommended.

✓ 12. **DO** . . . follow Step Two exercise guidelines.

step two

BREAKFAST

\+

LUNCH

▶ 2 glasses water prior to eating your lunch

\+

AFTERNOON SNACK

\+

DINNER

▶ Two glasses of water prior to eating your dinner

▶ Always begin dinner with either *LIFE* salad or *LIFE* soup

▶ No starch

SPECIAL NOTES

▶ Enjoy foods from Unlimited List any time throughout the day.

▶ All men and active women may eat unlimited protein portions at meals only.

▶ Enjoy one daily food from the *LIFE* Healthy Extra list.

in a nutshell

HOWARD DINOWITZ

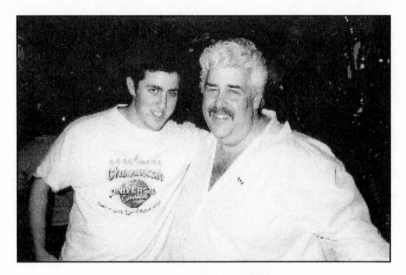

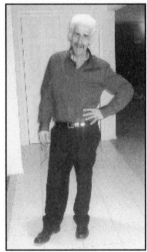

LOST: 219 pounds!

AGE: 50

HEIGHT: 5'10"

BEFORE: 388 pounds, size 60 waist

AFTER: 169 pounds, size 32 waist

THIN ACCOMPLISHMENTS: Having the energy to do everything I want to do . . . and I want to do everything!

THIN CHALLENGES: Now, my challenge is eating enough. If I skip meals, I can find myself getting a little light-headed. Who could have predicted that?

WORDS OF WISDOM: As a podiatrist, I know that weight is bad for the feet. So much of health is walking, and so much of walking is having good feet. The real devastating diseases sneak up and hit us around age 50. Taking off weight can help us—and our feet—stay healthier longer.

WHAT MADE YOU FINALLY DECIDE TO LOSE WEIGHT?
I was at a funeral, and when I tried to stand up to say a few words, I discovered that I was wedged in tight. I nearly broke the pew struggling out. I made a joke of it at the time, but I was terribly embarrassed.

WHAT PERSONAL RESOURCES HELPED YOU SUCCEED?
When I put my head to something, I do it all the way. That's what got me into this weight problem in the first place. When I ate, I *really* ate. But when I wanted to take the weight off, I got that done, too.

DID BEING A PHYSICIAN HELP YOU?
Only to the extent that I understood the downside of being fat. When you're at a healthy weight, your brain feels better. When your brain feels better, your body feels and works better. You sleep better, walk better, and can accomplish more.

AREN'T YOU EVER TEMPTED BY YOUR OLD FAVORITE FOODS?
I would be an idiot to choose to eat veal Parmesan with a bag of chips and a cold root beer when I could have something healthier and live longer. I'm too blessed, and I don't want to kick this blessing in the shins.

while). Snacks are interchangeable, too—as long as your choice is listed as an approved snack food.

Foods Allowed at Meals

(Wallet-sized printable lists of allowed foods for each step are available at www .JoyBauer.com)

Meats

Lean cuts only:

+ Bottom round
+ Buffalo
+ Filet mignon
+ Flank
+ London broil
+ Sirloin
+ Top round
+ Veal
+ Venison

Poultry (skinless only)

+ Chicken breast
+ Chicken breast, ground (at least 90% lean)
+ Chicken thigh
+ Cornish hen
+ Ostrich
+ **Poultry sausage (lean)**
+ **Turkey bacon**
+ Turkey breast
+ Turkey burger (lean)

- ✦ Turkey thigh
- ✦ Turkey, ground (at least 90% lean)

Pork

- ✦ **Ham, lean**
- ✦ Pork tenderloin

Fish and seafood

- ✦ Anchovies
- ✦ Catfish
- ✦ Clams
- ✦ Cod
- ✦ Crab (fresh, canned, or **imitation**)
- ✦ Flounder
- ✦ Haddock
- ✦ Halibut
- ✦ Lobster
- ✦ **Lox**
- ✦ Mackerel (Atlantic only, not king)
- ✦ Mahi mahi
- ✦ Mussels
- ✦ Oysters
- ✦ Red snapper
- ✦ Salmon, wild (fresh, canned, **or smoked**)
- ✦ Sardines
- ✦ Scallops
- ✦ Shrimp
- ✦ Sole
- ✦ Tilapia
- ✦ Trout
- ✦ Tuna (canned light in water)
- ✦ Whitefish

Eggs

- ✦ Egg whites
- ✦ Egg substitute
- ✦ **Eggs, whole (stick with noted amounts)**

Vegan Proteins

- ✦ Soy milk (low-fat)
- ✦ Soy yogurt (nonfat and low-fat)
- ✦ Tempeh
- ✦ Tofu
- ✦ Vegan cheese (nonfat and low-fat)
- ✦ Veggie burgers
- ✦ Wheat gluten/seitan

Dairy

- ✦ Cheese, fat-free (all varieties)
- ✦ Cheese, reduced-fat (all varieties)
- ✦ Cheese, Parmesan
- ✦ Cheese, Romano
- ✦ Greek yogurt (nonfat)
- ✦ **Yogurt, nonfat plain and flavored (all brands 100 calories or less per 6-ounce container)**

Vegetables (non-starchy only)

- ✦ Artichokes and artichoke hearts
- ✦ Asparagus
- ✦ Beans, non-starchy: green, yellow, Italian, and wax
- ✦ Beets
- ✦ Bok choy (Chinese cabbage)

BREAKFAST PROTEIN SUBSTITUTIONS

Beginning in Step Two, you have more options for protein with breakfast, and you gain the freedom to swap equivalent amounts of different proteins. Sometimes the substitution is obvious (such as swapping 5 ounces chicken for 5 ounces salmon), but other times it can be difficult to know exactly what makes for a good substitution. Here are some of my favorite breakfast suggestions, along with appropriate portion conversions.

INSTEAD OF . . .	TRY THIS!
1 hard boiled egg	*4 egg whites, hard boiled or scrambled—or-*
	3 slices turkey bacon—or-
	½ cup fat-free or 1% low-fat cottage cheese—or-
	1 cup skim milk or plain nonfat yogurt
3 slices turkey bacon	*one whole hard boiled egg or 4 egg whites—or-*
	½ cup fat-free or 1% low-fat cottage cheese—or-
	1 cup (8 oz) plain nonfat yogurt—or-
	6 ounces nonfat, flavored yogurt (any brand 100 calories or less)

✦ Broccoli

✦ Broccoli rabe

✦ Broccolini

✦ Brussels sprouts

✦ Cabbage

✦ Carrots

✦ Cauliflower

- ✦ Celery
- ✦ Dark green leafy vegetables:
    - ✦ Beet greens
    - ✦ Collard greens
    - ✦ Dandelion greens
    - ✦ Kale
    - ✦ Mustard greens
    - ✦ Spinach
    - ✦ Swiss chard
    - ✦ Turnip greens
- ✦ Eggplant
- ✦ Fennel
- ✦ Garlic
- ✦ Green onions (scallions)
- ✦ Jicama
- ✦ Leeks
- ✦ Lettuce:
    - ✦ Arugula
    - ✦ Endive
    - ✦ Escarole
    - ✦ Iceberg
    - ✦ Mixed greens/salad blends
    - ✦ Romaine
- ✦ Mixed vegetable blends without corn, starchy beans, peas, pasta, or any kind of sauce
- ✦ Mushrooms
- ✦ Okra
- ✦ Onion
- ✦ Peppers (all varieties)
- ✦ Pickles
- ✦ Pumpkin (fresh, frozen, or canned—must say "100% pure pumpkin," no sugar added)
- ✦ Radicchio

- Radishes
- Red peppers, roasted (if packed in oil, pat dry)
- Rhubarb
- **Sauerkraut**
- Sea vegetables (nori, etc.)
- Shallots
- Snow peas
- Spaghetti squash
- Sprouts (all varieties)
- Summer (yellow) squash
- Tomatoes
- Water chestnuts
- Watercress
- Zucchini

Starchy Vegetables

Starchy vegetables are part of Step Two menus *only* within specific breakfast and lunch recipes, and some afternoon snack options. Eat them only when designated at a particular meal—and carefully check your portions.

- **Beans (legumes)**
- **Green peas**
- **Lentils**
- **Sweet Potato**

Whole grains

Whole grains are incorporated into Step Two menus *only* within specific breakfast and lunch recipes, and some afternoon snack options. Eat whole grain items only when designated at a particular meal—and carefully check portions.

- *LIFE* Muffins (see recipes pages 119–123)
- Mini whole wheat pita bread (no more than 70 calories)
- **Regular whole wheat pita bread (no more than 150 calories)**
- Reduced calorie whole wheat bread (no more than 45 calories per slice)
- Rice cakes (stick with plain, 45 calories per rice cake)
- Wheat germ
- Whole grain bread (any brand that lists "whole wheat" as first ingredient)
- Whole grain cereal (any brand 150 calories or less per 1 cup serving; no more than 8 grams sugar; at least 3 grams fiber)
- **Whole grain English Muffin (any brand 130 calories or less)**
- Whole grain oats (plain flavor only; traditional, quick cooking or steel-cut oats)
- **Whole grain tortilla wrap (no more than 100 calories per wrap)**
- **Whole grain waffles (no more than 170 calories per 2 waffles)**

Fruit

Fruit is incorporated into Step Two menus *only* within specific breakfast, lunch, and dinner recipes, and some afternoon snack options. Eat fruit only when designated for a particular meal. Make careful note to eat only the amount listed—some meals list "HALF servings" and others list "WHOLE servings." (Note: When making substitutions, be sure to pick from the right serving size.)

HALF Fruit Serving Options
- Apple: 1 small (palm-sized)
- Apricot: 6 dried halves, or 3 whole (fresh or dried)
- Banana: ½ medium
- Berries: ¾ cup (fresh or frozen, unsweetened blueberries, raspberries, blackberries, boysenberries, or sliced strawberries; or 10 whole strawberries)
- Cantaloupe: ¼ medium or 1 cup cubed
- Cherries (fresh): ½ cup (about 10 whole)
- Clementines: 2

- ✦ Grapefruit: ½ (red, pink, or white)
- ✦ Grapes (seedless): ½ cup (red, purple, green, or black)
- ✦ Fruit salad: ½ cup fresh cut (from the produce section, unsweetened)
- ✦ Honeydew melon: 1 cup cubed
- ✦ Kiwi: 1 whole
- ✦ Mango: ½ fresh or ½ cup chunks (unsweetened)
- ✦ Nectarine: 1 whole
- ✦ Orange: 1 medium
- ✦ Papaya (fresh): 1 cup cubed
- ✦ Peach: 1 whole
- ✦ Pear: ½ large or 1 small
- ✦ Pineapple chunks (fresh): ½ cup
- ✦ Plum: 1 large
- ✦ Pomegranate: ½ medium
- ✦ Prunes: 3
- ✦ Raisins: 2 tablespoons
- ✦ Tangerine: 1 whole
- ✦ Watermelon, 1 cup cubed

WHOLE Fruit Serving Options

- ✦ Apple: 1 large
- ✦ Apricot: 12 dried halves, or 6 whole (fresh or dried)
- ✦ Banana: 1 whole
- ✦ Berries: 1½ cups (fresh or frozen, unsweetened blueberries, raspberries, blackberries, boysenberries, or sliced strawberries; or 20 whole strawberries)
- ✦ Cantaloupe: ½ medium or 2 cups cubed
- ✦ Cherries (fresh): 1 cup (about 20 whole)
- ✦ Clementines: 3
- ✦ Fruit salad: 1 cup fresh cut (from the produce section, unsweetened)
- ✦ Grapefruit: 1 whole (red, pink, or white)
- ✦ Grapes (seedless): 1 cup (red, purple, green, or black)
- ✦ Honeydew melon: 2 cups cubed
- ✦ Kiwi: 2 large

- Mango: 1 medium fresh or 1 cup chunks (unsweetened)
- Nectarines: 2
- Oranges: 2 medium
- Papaya (fresh): 2 cups cubed
- Peaches: 2 large
- Pear: 1 large
- Pineapple chunks: 1 cup fresh
- Plums: 2 large
- Pomegranate: 1 medium
- Prunes: 6
- Raisins: ¼ cup
- Tangerines: 2
- Watermelon: 2 cups cubed

Seasonings, Condiments, Marinades, and Healthy Fats

Your meal plans for Step Two make use of the following ingredients to flavor and jazz up your meals. Some of the condiments, such as vinegar, mustard, and hot sauce, are also included on the Unlimited List (see pages 41–42) and therefore can be added in unlimited quantities to ANY meal or snack, whether specified or not. For items not found on the Unlimited List, such as ketchup, mayo, and salad dressings, always stick with the portions designated in your meal plan.

- Avocado
- Chiles or hot peppers, fresh or canned in vinegar/water
- Extracts (vanilla, almond, peppermint, etc)
- **Fruit jam**
- **Honey**
- Horseradish
- Hot sauce
- Ketchup
- Lemon, fresh
- Lime, fresh

- **Maple syrup (real or reduced sugar/calorie)**
- Marinara sauce (opt for brands with 60 calories or less per ½ cup)
- Mayo reduced-fat (any brand, 25 calories or less per tablespoon)
- Mustard (plain, brown, spicy, Dijon)
- Nonstick cooking spray (any variety)
- Nuts (almonds, pistachios, walnuts, etc)
- Nut butters (peanut, soy, almond, etc.)
- Olive oil
- **Olives**
- **Orange juice, 100% juice**
- Salad dressing, Caesar (only use for Caesar salad lunch option—any brand, no more than 80 calories per 2 tablespoons)
- Salad dressing, low-calorie (any brand with no more than 40 calories per 2 tablespoons)
- Salad dressing, Joy's *LIFE* recipes (pages 60–63)
- Salsa (mild or spicy; any brand without added sugar or corn syrup)
- Salt substitute
- Soy sauce, low-sodium
- **Steak sauce**
- **Sugar, brown or white**
- Teriyaki sauce, low-sodium
- Vinegar, any type—not vinaigrette
- Wasabi
- **Worcestershire sauce**
- Herbs and Spices
    - Allspice
    - Anise seed
    - Basil
    - Bay leaves
    - Cardamom
    - Cayenne pepper
    - Celery seed
    - Chili powder

- Chinese five-spice
- Chives
- Cilantro
- Cinnamon
- Cloves
- Coriander
- Cumin
- Curry powder
- Dill weed
- Garlic powder
- Ginger
- Lemongrass
- Marjoram
- Mint
- Mustard
- Mustard seed
- Nutmeg
- Old Bay seasoning
- Onion powder
- Oregano
- Paprika
- Parsley
- Pepper (ground) and whole peppercorns
- Pumpkin pie spice
- Red pepper flakes
- Rosemary
- Sage
- Seasoning blends (without added sugar or salt)
- Tarragon
- Thyme
- Turmeric

Beverages

- Club soda
- Coffee (No added sugar, no artificial sweeteners, no cream or whole milk. You may add skim, 1%, or low-fat soy milk only.)
- Naturally flavored zero-calorie coffee with no sugar (see recipes on page 37)
- **Diet soda and other artificially sweetened beverages (each 12-ounce can or 20-ounce bottle counts as half of your daily artificial sweetener allotment)**
- Seltzer, zero calorie (plain and naturally flavored)
- Sparkling water
- Tea (black, white, green, herbal—no added sugar or honey; no added artificial sweeteners unless counted toward your daily allotment)
- Water
- Naturally flavored waters, calorie-free (see recipes, page 38)

ACCEPTABLE MID-AFTERNOON SNACK LIST (100–150 cal)

You may substitute afternoon snacks listed on your menu with the following options. Stick with one per day, and pay close attention to designated portions.

Cheese Options

- 1 ounce reduced-fat or fat-free cheese with unlimited celery and pepper sticks
- 1 ounce reduced-fat or fat-free cheese with 1 mini whole-grain pita (no more than 70 calories) or rice cake
- 1 ounce reduced-fat or fat-free cheese with 10 raw almonds or 15 pistachio nuts
- 1 part-skim cheese stick with a HALF fruit serving (see list)
- 4 level tablespoons reduced-fat cream cheese with unlimited celery sticks
- ½ cup low-fat or nonfat cottage cheese, topped with a HALF fruit serving
- ½ cup low-fat or nonfat cottage cheese with unlimited nonstarchy vegetables (i.e. cherry tomatoes, red pepper strips, celery, or baby carrots)

- ✦ ¾ cup low-fat or nonfat cottage cheese, plain or with cinnamon
- ✦ 1 slice reduced calorie, whole-grain toast (any brand 45 calories or less) with 1 ounce slice reduced or nonfat cheese and optional tomato slices
- ✦ 1 slice reduced calorie, whole-grain toast (any brand, 45 calories or less per slice) with 1 level tablespoon reduced-fat cream cheese

Yogurt Options

- ✦ **8 ounces nonfat plain, Greek, or any flavored yogurt (150 calories or less)**
- ✦ **6 ounces nonfat plain, Greek, or any flavored yogurt (100 calories or less), topped with 2 tablespoons wheat germ or ground flaxseed**
- ✦ **6 ounces nonfat plain, Greek, or any flavored yogurt (100 calories or less), topped with a HALF fruit serving**
- ✦ **Vanilla Pumpkin Pudding: 6 ounces nonfat vanilla yogurt (any brand, 100 calories or less) mixed with ½ cup 100-percent pure pumpkin puree and cinnamon to taste**

Nut and Nut Butter Options

- ✦ 10 raw almonds or 15 pistachios and a HALF fruit serving
- ✦ 10 raw almonds or 15 pistachios and ½ cup (one snack container) no-sugar-added natural applesauce
- ✦ 20 raw almonds
- ✦ 30 pistachios
- ✦ 2 level teaspoons natural peanut butter and a HALF fruit serving, e.g., ½ banana or 1 small apple
- ✦ 1 level tablespoon natural peanut butter with unlimited celery sticks
- ✦ 1 slice reduced calorie, whole-grain toast (any brand, 45 calories or less per slice) with 1 level tablespoon natural peanut butter

Fruit Options

- ✦ 1 frozen banana
- ✦ 1 cup frozen grapes
- ✦ One WHOLE fruit serving

- 1 orange (or any other HALF fruit serving) and 1 mini whole-grain pita (no more than 70 calories)
- **1 LIFE Smoothie (see recipe pages 132–133)**

Miscellaneous Options

- 4 ounces turkey breast rolled with lettuce and mustard
- 1 mini whole-grain pita (no more than 70 calories) with 2 level tablespoons hummus (any variety)
- ¼ cup hummus (any variety) with unlimited cucumber slices, celery sticks, and/or red, yellow, and green bell pepper strips
- 1 cup edamame beans boiled in the pod (green soybeans, fresh or frozen)
- **½ medium ripe avocado drizzled with lime juice, salt and pepper to taste**
- **1 rice cake + one hard boiled egg (or 4 egg whites)**
- **1 slice reduced-calorie, whole-grain toast (any brand, 45 calories or less per slice) topped with one hard boiled egg mashed and mixed with minced onion and 1 teaspoon reduced-fat mayonnaise.**
- **1 *LIFE* Muffin (see recipe on pages 119–123)**
- **1 Joy Bauer *LIFE* Bar**

UNLIMITED FOOD/BEVERAGE LIST

Enjoy in unlimited amounts—at any time of the day.

- ALL non-starchy vegetables! (see vegetables list on pages 29–31)
- Club soda (with optional fresh lemon or lime)
- Coffee (black, or with skim, 1%, or soy milk only; no sugar)
- Naturally flavored zero-calorie coffee with no sugar (see recipes on page 37)
- Extracts (vanilla, almond, peppermint, etc.)
- Herbs and spices (see list on pages 35–36)
- Horseradish
- Hot sauce
- Lemon and lime wedges

- Low-sodium broth
- Mustard (plain, brown, spicy, Dijon)
- Nonstick cooking spray
- Joy's *LIFE* Balsamic Vinaigrette Salad Dressing
- **Salsa (mild or spicy; any brand without added sugar or corn syrup)**
- Salt substitute
- Seltzer water (plain or naturally flavored with optional fresh lemon or lime)
- Sparkling water
- **Soy sauce, low-sodium**
- Tea (iced or hot, with lemon or skim, 1%, or soy milk only; no sugar or honey)
- Vinegar (any variety)
- Wasabi
- Water (with optional fresh lemon or lime)
- Naturally flavored waters, zero calorie (see recipe, page 38)
- **Worcestershire sauce**

JANICE MIELARCZYK

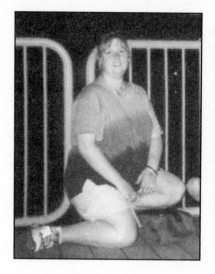 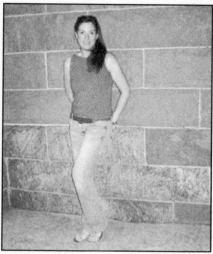

LOST: 75 pounds!

AGE: 40

HEIGHT: 5'5"

BEFORE: 205 pounds, size 20/22

AFTER: 130 pounds, size 6

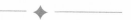

THIN ACCOMPLISHMENTS: I run! I kayak! I do spinning classes! I was never athletic—my personal motto had always been: *I don't sweat on purpose.* I enjoy activity so much now. I have found the natural rhythm and weight of my body.

THIN CHALLENGES: I love food. I know everyone says that, but I really love food. Eating was the focal point of all our social occasions. But I tell myself that I can either eat what I want *or* wear what I want. My new motto is: *Donna Karan, Vera Wang.*

WORDS OF WISDOM: Everyone wants to know how long it's going to take. Time is going to go by no matter what, why not work toward thin?

DID WEIGHT LOSS COME EASY FOR YOU?

Not nearly. I hit the 200 mark before I realized I had to lose about 60 pounds. 60! It was more than I thought I could handle. Still, I dieted for a full week—barely ate anything, or so I thought—except at night, when I ate everything. Still, it felt like suffering. At the end of that week, I had *gained* a pound.

HOW DID YOU RECOVER FROM THAT?

I had to rethink what I was doing. Instead of trying to lose 61 pounds, I concentrated on losing 1 pound. At least I'd be back in the same position as a week earlier. *That* seemed reasonable. With that in mind, I ended up losing 4 pounds the next week. After that, my goal was to lose just one pound per week.

DO YOU HAVE ANY WEIGHT LOSS TRICKS?

I keep a food journal for a week each month. When I was actively losing weight, I kept the journal every day. But by now, I know what I'm doing. But I don't want to get too comfortable with the process, slip up, and put the weight back on. Now I weigh myself daily, but I journal one week a month to keep myself in line.

ON THE WEIGHT LOSS STRUGGLE . . .

When I weighed 205, I had physical weight *and* mental weight—how I felt, the lack of energy, what people thought of me. Healthy weight means making choices everyday, but the more often you make the right choice, the easier it becomes. I lost weight to look better, but I maintain the loss because it feels so good.

JOY'S LESSONS LEARNED

THE CHOICE IS YOURS: *Although it can be tough (and frustrating) to watch what you eat, it's certainly tough and even **more** frustrating to feel heavy and sluggish.*

Step Two
Menus and Recipes

On the following pages are meal plans for the full 14 days of Step Two.

Feel free to repeat or swap corresponding meals—breakfast for breakfast, lunch for lunch, or dinner for dinner (from among Step Two or Step One meals *only*).

If you're a member of the online program at www.JoyBauer.com, you'll be able to browse even more Step Two meals and recipes. For a list of the easiest, low-prep meals for Step Two, see pages 115–116.

In the event that you must eat out during the next two weeks, follow my LIFE Diet Step Two Restaurant Options on pages 116–119.

Special Instructions for All Men and Some Active Women
(Follow these instructions if you are a man, or if you are a woman under age 40 who does more than one hour of cardiovascular exercise at least 6 days each week.) Although specific portions are listed for protein at each meal (egg whites, meat, chicken, turkey, fish and seafood, tofu), all men and active women may eat *unlimited* protein portions at meals only—that means breakfast, lunch, and dinner, but not with your snack or throughout the rest of the day.

Special Instructions for Vegetarians
Substitute low-fat soy milk, soy yogurt, and soy cheese for dairy products. For meat and poultry, substitute an equivalent portion of fish, seafood, tempeh, or meat analog products. If opting to replace meat with tofu, double the portion size listed (since tofu is less dense than meat). You may also substitute veggie burgers for turkey burgers or other meat entrées.

LIFE Healthy Extra
Enjoy *one per day* from approved food list (pages 75–76).

BREAKFAST

LIFE Muffin* (pages 119–123) with Hard Boiled Egg

> ** May enjoy any LIFE muffin recipe: Apple Cinnamon Muffin, Mango Ginger Muffin, Carrot Spice Muffin, Dark Chocolate Cherry Muffin, Banana Blueberry Muffin*

LUNCH

Curried Chicken Salad with Sweet Green Peas (page 127)

Unlimited Crunchy Celery and Pepper Sticks

SNACK

Fruit & Nuts

> *Any HALF serving of fruit +10 raw almonds or 15 pistachios*

DINNER

LIFE Dinner Salad (page 59)

~ or ~

2 cups *LIFE* Veggie Soup (page 63)

Sirloin Steak with Creamy Horseradish Sauce (page 63)

> *5 ounces lean sirloin steak, seasoned as desired. Preheat a large skillet or grill to medium-high heat and cook to preferred temperature.*
>
> *Top with mixture of 1 heaping tablespoon low-fat or nonfat sour cream and 1 teaspoon horseradish.*

Parmesan Broiled Tomato (page 142)

BREAKFAST

English Muffin with Cream Cheese, Tomato, and Lox

Opened-faced, toasted whole-grain English muffin (any brand 130 calories or less) with 2 tablespoons reduced-fat or fat-free cream cheese (one tablespoon per slice), unlimited sliced tomato, and 2 ounces sliced lox (one ounce for each slice). Can use 2 slices reduced-calorie whole wheat toast (45 calories or less per slice) instead of English muffin. Add sliced onion if desired.

LUNCH

Turkey Burger on Greens

5-ounce turkey burger (page 68) on a bed of mixed greens or spinach (unlimited amounts) with lettuce, tomato, onion, and/or pickle

2 tablespoons ketchup or salsa (optional)

Raw or steamed vegetables

Your choice of unlimited amounts approved veggies

SNACK

1 part-skim cheese stick with HALF fruit serving

DINNER

LIFE Dinner Salad (page 59)

~ or ~

2 cups *LIFE* Veggie Soup (page 63)
Chicken Florentine (page 140)

BREAKFAST
Sweet Potato Skillet (page 124)

LUNCH
Veggie Tuna Salad (page 127) over Spinach Leaves
~and~
2 Rice Cakes and Tomato slices

SNACK
LIFE Muffin
>   *Any flavor (pages 119–123)*

DINNER
LIFE Dinner Salad (page 59)
~ or ~
2 cups *LIFE* Veggie Soup (page 63)
Tandoori Halibut Kebabs (page 141)
Sweet and Sour Cucumber Salad
>   *Thinly slice half a cucumber (peeled) and half a red bell pepper. In a small*
>   *bowl, whisk together 1 teaspoon honey, 1 to 2 tablespoons unsweetened rice*
>   *wine or cider vinegar, pinch of salt, and 1 tablespoon chopped fresh mint*
>   *(optional). Add dressing to vegetables and toss to coat.*

BREAKFAST

Whole Grain Waffles with Yogurt

2 frozen whole grain waffles, toasted (any brand, 170 calories or less per two waffles) with 6 ounces plain or nonfat flavored yogurt (100 calories or less per 6 ounces container) or ½ cup 1% low-fat cottage cheese

LUNCH

Chicken-Apple Salad Chop (page 128)

SNACK

One rice cake + one hard boiled egg (or 4 to 5 egg whites)

DINNER

LIFE Dinner Salad (page 59)

~ or ~

2 cups *LIFE* Veggie Soup (page 63)

Turkey Sausage with Sautéed Peppers and Onion (page 144)

BREAKFAST

Creamy Scrambled Eggs with Chives and Turkey Bacon

> *In bowl, beat together 1 whole large egg and 3 egg whites, 2 tablespoons reduced-fat or nonfat sour cream or nonfat cream cheese, and 1 to 2 tablespoons minced scallions or chives.*
>
> *Cook over medium heat in heated pan coated with nonstick cooking spray.*
>
> *Serve with 2 slices reduced-fat turkey bacon.*

LUNCH

Whole Wheat Pita Pizza (page 128)

SNACK

> *One WHOLE fruit serving (see list pages 166–167)*

DINNER

LIFE Dinner Salad (page 59)

~ or ~

2 cups *LIFE* Veggie Soup (page 63)

Orange Dijon Pork Tenderloin (page 144)

Steamed green beans or sugar snap peas

> *Unlimited*

BREAKFAST

Pumpkin Oatmeal

Prepare ½ cup dry instant oatmeal with water as directed.

Combine cooked oatmeal with 1 teaspoon vanilla extract, ½ cup canned 100% pure pumpkin puree, dash cinnamon (optional), and 2 to 3 teaspoons sugar or artificial sweetener (optional).

LUNCH

Stuffed Vegetable Omelet (page 129)

~ plus ~

Whole Grain English Muffin

One dry toasted

SNACK

¾ cup low-fat or nonfat cottage cheese, plain or with cinnamon

DINNER

LIFE Dinner Salad (page 59)

~ or ~

2 cups *LIFE* Veggie Soup (page 63)

Honey Mustard Chicken

Mix together 2 tablespoons Dijon mustard, 2 teaspoons honey, and black pepper to taste. Pan sauté (with nonstick cooking spray) or grill 5 ounce boneless, skinless chicken breast. Five minutes before the end of cooking, brush with half of the honey mustard mixture. Serve; use the remaining honey mustard as a dip for chicken.

Roasted Balsamic Asparagus

Preheat oven to 350°F. Assemble the asparagus on a baking sheet sprayed with nonstick cooking spray.

Drizzle the asparagus with 1 to 2 tablespoons balsamic vinegar and season with salt and pepper to taste.

Roast for 20 minutes.

BREAKFAST

Broiled Grapefruit with Cottage Cheese

Cut 1 whole grapefruit in half. Sprinkle each half with 1 teaspoon brown or granulated sugar (optional). Place under a preheated broiler until bubbly, about 3 to 5 minutes.

Enjoy with ½ cup 1% low-fat or nonfat cottage cheese on side.

LUNCH

Thanksgiving Turkey Sandwich

Spread 2 slices lightly toasted, reduced-calorie whole wheat bread with 2 tablespoons reduced-fat or nonfat cream cheese (1 tablespoon per slice).

Top with 4 ounces turkey breast, arugula, spinach, or romaine lettuce, and 1 tablespoon "whole berry" cranberry sauce.

Baby Carrots

unlimited

SNACK

6 ounces nonfat plain, Greek, or flavored yogurt (any brand 100 calories or less)

+ HALF serving fruit (see list pages 32–33)

DINNER

LIFE Dinner Salad (page 59)

~ or ~

2 cups *LIFE* Veggie Soup (page 63)
Chesapeake Shrimp Boil (page 138)
Stewed Okra and Tomatoes (page 138)

(or, unlimited steamed zucchini, summer squash, okra, or green beans)

BREAKFAST

LIFE Smoothie (pages 132–133)

> *Choose from Banana Cardamom, Blueberry Mango, Creamsicle, or Strawberry Banana Smoothie*

~plus~

Turkey Bacon

> *3 slices*

LUNCH

Open Faced Tuna Melt (page 130)

SNACK

> *4 ounces turkey breast rolled with lettuce and mustard*

DINNER

LIFE Dinner Salad (page 59)

~ or ~

2 cups *LIFE* Veggie Soup (page 63)

LIFE Quiche (page 137)

BREAKFAST

Apple Cinnamon Pancakes with Yogurt Topping (pages 124–125)

LUNCH

Wild Salmon Salad with Mixed Greens

6-ounces of canned wild salmon (boneless, skinless) mashed with 1 table-spoon reduced-fat mayo, 1 to 2 teaspoons Dijon mustard, minced onion (optional), ½ teaspoon optional Worcestershire sauce, and black pepper to taste.

Serve over mixed greens with 2 to 4 tablespoons low-calorie dressing (or one teaspoon olive oil and unlimited vinegar or lemon)

SNACK

Natural peanut butter (1 level tablespoon) with unlimited celery sticks

DINNER

LIFE Dinner Salad (page 59)

~ or ~

2 cups *LIFE* Veggie Soup (page 63)
Easy Chicken Puttanesca (page 139)

BREAKFAST

Breakfast BLT

Whole grain English muffin, toasted (any brand 130 calories or less)

3 slices lean turkey bacon, tomato slices, lettuce leaves, and

1 tablespoon reduced-fat mayo

LUNCH

Cottage Cheese and Fruit

1 cup fat-free or 1% low-fat cottage cheese plus

one WHOLE fruit serving plus

your choice of 1 tablespoon chopped nuts or 2 tablespoons ground flaxseed or 2 tablespoons wheat germ

SNACK

One rice cake+one hard boiled egg (or four egg whites)

DINNER

LIFE Dinner Salad (page 59)

~ or ~

2 cups *LIFE* Veggie Soup (page 63)
LIFE Shepherd's Pie (page 143)

BREAKFAST

Ham and Cheese Omelet with Chives (page 126)

LUNCH

Mediterranean Pita with Tomato Cucumber Salad

> *2 mini whole wheat pita*
>
> *¼ cup hummus, divided*
>
> *Lettuce, tomato, cucumber, bean sprouts, shredded carrot*
>
> *Enjoy with unlimited chopped cucumber, tomato, and red onion drizzled with one teaspoon olive oil and red wine vinegar; season with ground pepper, salt, and oregano to taste.*

SNACK

> *One LIFE Muffin (any flavor, pages 119–123)*

DINNER

LIFE Dinner Salad (page 59)

~ or ~

2 cups *LIFE* Veggie Soup (page 63)

Grilled Sirloin Steak

> *5 ounces lean steak, seasoned as desired with allowed marinades/herbs/ seasonings.*
>
> *Preheat a large skillet or grill to medium-high heat and cook to preferred temperature.*

E-Z Garlic Broccoli

> *Preheat oven to 450°F. Cut one large bunch of broccoli into florets.*
>
> *Sprinkle with 1 clove minced garlic (1 teaspoon) and season with salt and pepper.*
>
> *Tightly wrap in aluminum foil and place in oven for 8 to 10 minutes.*

BREAKFAST

Apple Slices with Peanut Butter

One sliced apple with 2 level tablespoons natural peanut butter

LUNCH

Turkey Tortilla Roll Up (page 129)

Unlimited crunchy pepper and celery sticks

SNACK

20 raw almonds or 30 pistachio nuts

DINNER

LIFE Dinner Salad (page 59)

~ or ~

2 cups *LIFE* Veggie Soup (page 63)

Shrimp Ceviche with Lime (page 142)

BREAKFASTS

Whole Grain Waffles with Yogurt (Day 4)

> *Bonus Timesaver: Cut toasted waffles into strips and dip into a 6 ounce yogurt container to eat on the go.*

Broiled Grapefruit with Cottage Cheese (Day 7)

> *Bonus Timesaver: Skip the broiling step and enjoy your grapefruit fresh (or select any other HALF fruit serving).*

Apple Slices with Peanut Butter (Day 12)

LIFE Oatmeal Pancake (Day 14)

LUNCHES

Open Faced Tuna Melt (Day 8)

> *Bonus Timesaver: Top cold tuna salad with a tomato slice and leave off cheese.*

Wild Salmon Salad with Mixed Green Salad (Day 9)

> *Bonus Timesaver: For your salad, enjoy a few handfuls of any lettuce blend directly out of the sack. No need to add anything else!*

Cottage Cheese and Fruit (Day 10)

Turkey Tortilla Roll Up (Day 12)

> *Bonus Timesaver: For your side veggies, use baby carrots straight from the bag.*

Lentil Soup and Salad (Day 13)

> *Bonus Timesaver: Use store bought soup (any brand 300 calories or less per two cup serving). For your salad, enjoy a few handfuls of any lettuce blend directly out of the sack. No need to add anything else!*

DINNERS

LIFE Salad (every day)

> *Bonus Timesaver: Open a pre-washed bag of salad and drizzle on low-cal dressing or plain balsamic vinegar.*

(Continued)

easiest meals at-a-glance

step two

Sirloin Steak with Creamy Horseradish Sauce with Parmesan Broiled Tomato
(Day 1)

> *Bonus Timesaver: Use 2 tablespoons ketchup or steak sauce in place of
> horseradish sauce, or enjoy your steak plain. Skip the* **Parmesan Broiled
> Tomato** *and enjoy any nonstarchy vegetable in your fridge or freezer.*

Turkey Sausage with Sautéed Peppers and Onions (Day 4)

Orange Dijon Pork Tenderloin with Steamed Vegetables (Day 5)

Honey Mustard Chicken with Balsamic Asparagus (Day 6)

> *Bonus Timesaver: Skip the* **Balsamic Asparagus** *recipe and instead simply
> microwave your asparagus (add salt, pepper, and preferred seasonings to
> taste).*

Grilled Sirloin Steak with EZ Garlic Broccoli (Day 11)

> *Bonus Timesaver: Skip the EZ Garlic Broccoli recipe and microwave plain
> broccoli or cauliflower (salt and pepper to taste).*

Baked Tilapia or Wild Salmon with Sautéed Spinach (Day 14)

> *Bonus Timesaver: Microwave a box of frozen chopped spinach (salt and
> pepper to taste) in place of sautéed spinach.*

easiest meals at-a-glance

Joy's LIFE Diet Step Two Restaurant Options

Some Step Two menu options can easily be ordered in a restaurant, as long as you
are willing to make a few special requests about how the foods are prepared. But
there are also some generic meals you can order anytime and nearly anywhere.

(Always remember: If it is not listed here or in the Unlimited Foods list, don't eat it! For example, don't eat extra bread, rice, fruit, full-fat salad dressings, sauces, etc.)

Breakfast

Option #1: Egg white omelet stuffed with any of your favorite vegetables (no cheese—most restaurants don't carry reduced-fat cheese), plus ½ grapefruit or ¼ cantaloupe, or side portion of fresh berries or fruit salad.

Option #2: One hard boiled egg with one cup plain oatmeal. Top oatmeal with a few tablespoons of berries *or* 1 teaspoon/packet sugar. Artificial sweetener is optional.

Option #3: Scrambled egg whites with optional chopped tomatoes and herbs + one slice whole wheat toast, dry.

For all options, add beverage: Coffee (black, or with skim or 1% milk only) or tea (iced or hot, unsweetened, with lemon *or* skim or 1% milk only).

Lunch

Option #1: Large salad piled with assorted raw vegetables and topped with skinless grilled chicken *or* turkey *or* fish/seafood (no cheese). Use plain balsamic vinegar or fresh lemon as dressing, or 2 tablespoons low-calorie dressing (if available).

Option #2: Turkey burger, no bun, with lettuce, tomato, onion, pickles, and optional ketchup and/or mustard. Enjoy your burger with plain raw or steamed vegetables. Or, with a vegetable salad dressed with plain vinegar or fresh lemon.

Option #3: Turkey sandwich on ONE slice whole wheat bread (remove top slice)—enjoy with any of the following toppings; lettuce, tomato, roasted peppers, onion, pickles and mustard.

Option #4: One bowl of any non-creamy vegetable-based soup (lentil, black bean, or vegetable) along with a plain mixed vegetable salad (omit cheese, croutons, and other high calorie salad ingredients). Dress the salad with vinegar, fresh lemon or 2 tablespoons low-calorie dressing.

For all options, add beverage: Water, seltzer, coffee (black, or with skim or 1% milk only), and/or tea (iced or hot, unsweetened, with lemon or skim or 1% milk only)

Dinner

OPTION #1: STANDARD RESTAURANT

House salad with plain vinegar or fresh lemon.

Skinless chicken breast *or* fish *or* seafood *or* pork tenderloin *or* turkey *or* lean steak (all options must be grilled, baked, roasted, poached, steamed, or boiled *only*).

Double order of steamed, plain vegetables.

OPTION #2: STEAK HOUSE

Sliced tomatoes and onion with plain balsamic vinegar (*not* balsamic "vinaigrette")

Shrimp cocktail with cocktail sauce and lemon

Grilled or broiled lean steak (sirloin or filet mignon are good options)

Steamed broccoli, spinach, or green beans (add lemon, salt, and pepper to taste)

OPTION #3: CHINESE FOOD

Cup of soup (choose either egg drop or hot and sour soup or wonton broth without wontons or noodles)

Order "steamed" chicken, shrimp, or tofu with vegetables. Request garlic sauce on the side and drizzle ONLY one tablespoon on your steamed entrée (you may add additional low-sodium soy sauce). Avoid all extras including rice, dumplings, noodles, wontons, etc.

OPTION #4: JAPANESE FOOD (2 CHOICES)

Teriyaki Dinner:

Miso soup + Chicken or Salmon Teriyaki with Vegetables. Omit the rice and ask the waiter to double up on vegetables.

Sashimi Dinner:

Miso soup + unlimited sashimi (fish *without* the rice) + (optional ginger, wasabi, and soy sauce) + side order of steamed vegetables topped with low-sodium soy sauce or fresh lemon.

For all options, add beverage: Water, seltzer, tea (iced or hot, unsweetened, with lemon *or* skim or 1% milk only). Great after-dinner choices include all herbal teas (especially mint or chamomile) and green tea.

Recipes—Breakfasts

LIFE APPLE CINNAMON MUFFINS

½ cup applesauce, unsweetened

½ cup skim milk

½ cup nonfat plain yogurt

4 egg whites

1 teaspoon vanilla

½ cup brown sugar

1 teaspoon baking powder

1 teaspoon baking soda

1½ teaspoons cinnamon

½ teaspoon nutmeg

¼ teaspoon salt

2 cups whole wheat flour

2 cups peeled, finely cubed apples (preferably Granny Smith)

Preheat the oven to 350°F. Prepare the muffin pan with muffin liners and spray with nonstick spray. In a large bowl, mix together the applesauce, milk, yogurt, egg whites, and vanilla. Add the sugar, baking powder, baking soda, cinnamon, nutmeg, and salt, and stir to combine. Sprinkle flour over the batter and fold together delicately, making sure to not over-mix. Fold in apples. Spoon batter into muffin cups. Bake for approximately 20 to 25 minutes, or until an inserted tooth-pick comes out clean. The muffins can be frozen in an air-tight container, sealed freezer bag, or individually wrapped for up to 2 months. For best results, freeze muffins immediately after baking and cooling to room temperature.

Makes 12 muffins

LIFE MANGO GINGER MUFFINS

½ cup applesauce, unsweetened

½ cup skim milk

½ cup nonfat plain yogurt

4 egg whites

1 teaspoon vanilla

½ cup brown sugar

1 teaspoon baking powder

1 teaspoon baking soda

1½ teaspoons ground ginger (or 1 teaspoon fresh ginger, minced or grated)

¼ teaspoon salt

2 cups whole wheat flour

2 cups peeled, finely cubed mango (use a slightly firm mango for best results)

Preheat oven to 350°F. Prepare muffin pan with muffin liners and spray with non-stick spray. In a large bowl, mix together the applesauce, milk, yogurt, egg whites, and vanilla. Add the sugar, baking powder, baking soda, ginger, and salt, and stir to combine. Sprinkle flour over the batter and fold together delicately, making sure not to over-mix. Fold in the mango. Spoon the batter into muffin cups. Bake for approximately 20 to 25 minutes, or until an inserted toothpick comes out clean. The muffins can be frozen in an air-tight container, sealed freezer bag, or individually wrapped for up to 2 months. For best results, freeze muffins immediately after baking and cooling to room temperature.

Makes 12 muffins

LIFE CARROT SPICE MUFFINS

1 cup all-purpose flour

½ cup whole wheat flour

¼ cup granulated sugar

1 teaspoon baking powder

1 teaspoon baking soda

2 tablespoons ground flaxseed

1 teaspoon ground cinnamon

1 teaspoon ground ginger

½ teaspoon ground nutmeg

1 teaspoon salt

1½ cups peeled, shredded carrot

⅓ cup pitted, chopped dates or raisins

½ cup unsweetened apple sauce

½ cup fat-free plain yogurt

¼ cup water

1 teaspoon vanilla extract

2 large egg whites

¼ cup honey

Preheat oven to 375°F. Prepare muffin pan with muffin liners and spray with non-stick spray. In a large bowl, combine all the dry ingredients and stir to combine. Add the shredded carrots and chopped dates and stir to thoroughly coat. In another bowl, combine the wet ingredients: apple sauce, yogurt, water, vanilla, egg whites, and honey. Whisk until combined. Add the wet ingredients to the flour/carrot/date mixture and stir using a wooden spoon. The batter will be thick. Spoon the batter into the muffin cups and bake at 375°F for 20 minutes, or until an inserted tooth-pick comes out clean.

The muffins can be frozen in an air-tight container, sealed freezer bag, or individually wrapped for up to 2 months. For best results, freeze muffins immediately after baking and cooling to room temperature.

Makes 12 muffins

LIFE DARK CHOCOLATE CHERRY MUFFINS

½ cup plus 1 tablespoon real maple syrup

½ cup unsweetened apple sauce

¾ cup fat-free milk

1 tablespoon strong coffee

3 large egg whites

¾ cup fat-free vanilla yogurt

1 teaspoon vanilla

1½ cups whole wheat flour

½ teaspoon salt

1 teaspoon baking powder

1 teaspoon baking soda

6 tablespoons unsweetened cocoa powder

⅔ cup dried cherries

Heat oven to 325°F. Prepare muffin pan with muffin liners and spray with non-stick spray. Combine dry ingredients in a large mixing bowl. In a separate bowl, combine the wet ingredients: maple syrup, apple sauce, milk, coffee, vanilla, egg whites, and yogurt. Add the wet ingredients to the dry ingredients and stir well to combine. Stir in the cherries. Fill the muffin cups ¾ full with batter. Bake at 325°F for 20 to 25 minutes, or until an inserted toothpick comes out clean. The muffins can be frozen in an air-tight container, sealed freezer bag, or individually wrapped for up to 2 months. For best results, freeze muffins immediately after baking and cooling to room temperature.

Makes 12 muffins

LIFE BANANA BLUEBERRY MUFFINS

2 tablespoons fat-free sour cream

2 tablespoons low-fat buttermilk

1 large egg

⅓ cup whole wheat flour

½ cup oat bran

¾ teaspoon baking powder

¾ teaspoon baking soda

¼ teaspoon salt

1½ cups mashed banana (approximately 3 medium ripe bananas)

2 tablespoons brown sugar

½ cup blueberries, fresh or frozen, unsweetened

½ teaspoon grated orange zest (optional)

Preheat oven to 375°F. Spray a standard muffin pan with nonstick cooking spray. In a medium bowl, whisk together the sour cream, buttermilk, and egg. In a second bowl, stir together the flour, oat bran, baking powder, baking soda, and salt. In a third, large bowl, mash bananas with a fork, potato masher, or your hands. Fold the sugar into the mashed banana. Add the buttermilk mixture and combine well. Sprinkle the flour mixture over the banana mixture, fold to combine, being sure not to over-mix. Gently fold in the blueberries and orange zest. Spoon the batter into muffin cups filling ¾ of the way. Bake at 375°F for 15 to 20 minutes, or until an inserted toothpick comes out clean. The muffins can be frozen in an air-tight container, sealed freezer bag, or individually wrapped for up to 2 months. For best results, freeze muffins immediately after baking and cooling to room temperature.

Makes 6 muffins

SWEET POTATO SKILLET

½ medium sweet potato (6 ounces)

½ to ¾ cup diced bell pepper and onion

½ teaspoon paprika

Salt and pepper to taste

1 ounce low-fat or nonfat cheese, shredded or sliced thin

1 tablespoon fresh parsley, chopped (optional)

Peel sweet potato and prick with a fork, wrap in dampened paper towel, and microwave for 3 to 5 minutes. Allow to cool for 5 minutes before dicing. Meanwhile, heat a nonstick pan to medium high. Spray with cooking spray, then add the peppers and onions and sauté for 5 to 7 minutes or until tender. Add the diced sweet potato and sauté for an additional 3 to 5 minutes until all the veggies are tender and lightly browned. Transfer them to a plate and top with the cheese and parsley.

Makes one serving

APPLE CINNAMON PANCAKES WITH YOGURT TOPPING

Pancakes

1 cup whole wheat flour

1 cup fat-free milk

1 egg white

¼ cup fat-free vanilla yogurt

1 tablespoon honey

2 teaspoons vanilla extract

1 teaspoon ground cinnamon

⅛ teaspoon nutmeg

½ teaspoon baking soda

1 cup diced peeled apple, preferably Golden Delicious

Topping

8 ounces nonfat flavored yogurt (any preferred flavor, such as lemon, vanilla or strawberry)

Combine the flour, milk, egg white, yogurt, honey, vanilla, cinnamon, nutmeg, and baking soda in a blender and blend until smooth, or thoroughly mix ingredients by hand. Stir in the apple. Spray a griddle or large fry pan with nonstick cooking spray. When pan is hot, ladle about 2 tablespoons of batter onto the griddle for each pancake. Cook until small bubbles form around the edges, 1 to 2 minutes. Flip the pancakes, and cook about 1 minute longer, until the centers are cooked through and outsides are golden brown. Serve immediately with the fat-free yogurt topping of choice, or allow to cool and freeze in an air-tight container. Note: One serving=3 pancakes with a *total* of ¼ cup (2 rounded tablespoons) yogurt topping.

Makes 4 servings, 3 pancakes and ¼ cup nonfat yogurt topping each

BREAKFAST PIZZA

1 whole egg and 2 egg whites

Mini whole wheat pita

1 tablespoon plus 1 tablespoon reduced-fat (part-skim) mozzarella cheese

Hot sauce (optional)

2 tablespoons salsa (optional)

Scramble the eggs in a pan coated with nonstick spray over medium heat.

Split the pita crosswise to form two rounds. Top each round with half the scrambled egg mixture and 1 tablespoon mozzarella.

Broil until the cheese is hot and bubbly.

Remove from the oven and top with the salsa and hot sauce.

Makes one serving

HAM AND CHEESE OMELET WITH CHIVES

1 whole large egg and 3 egg whites

Minced chives

2 ounces sliced or shredded lean ham

Preferred seasonings

2 tablespoons reduced-fat cheese

Preheat a pan coated with nonstick cooking spray over medium heat. Whip the eggs with the chives and pour into the pan. Sprinkle in the ham. Add the seasonings and continue to cook. When the bottom side is cooked, gently flip and cook the other side. Add the cheese and fold one side over the other.

Makes one serving

LIFE OATMEAL PANCAKE

½ cup quick-cooking (plain) oatmeal, dry (do not use steel cut oats)

4 egg whites, whipped

½ teaspoon ground cinnamon (optional)

½ teaspoon vanilla extract

1 tablespoon granulated sugar

Thoroughly whip together the oatmeal, egg whites, cinnamon, vanilla, and sugar. Preheat a pan coated with nonstick cooking spray over medium heat. Pour in the batter and cook for 2 to 3 minutes (for a moister pancake, cover the pan with a lid while cooking). When golden brown, flip and cook the other side. (This prepares one large pancake; you may choose to make 2 to 3 small pancakes instead.)

Makes one serving

CURRIED CHICKEN SALAD WITH SWEET GREEN PEAS

½ cup frozen green peas*

4 ounces cooked chicken breast, shredded or chopped (canned or fresh)

1 tablespoon reduced-fat mayo

1 to 3 tablespoons minced onion

1 teaspoon curry powder

Salad greens

*1 teaspoon olive oil with unlimited plain vinegar or fresh lemon (or 2 tablespoons
reduced calorie salad dressing)*

*For a sweeter salad, use ½ cup diced green or red grapes in place of green peas.

Rinse the green peas in a colander under cold water until thawed. Mash the chicken breast and gently mix with mayo, onion, curry powder, and peas. Serve over salad greens with preferred dressing.

Makes one serving

VEGGIE TUNA SALAD

1 can (6 ounces) chunk light tuna in water, drained

½ carrot, peeled and diced

½ celery stalk, diced

¼ red pepper, diced

¼ yellow pepper, diced

½ scallion, minced

1 tablespoon reduced-fat mayonnaise

½ teaspoon lemon juice

In a medium bowl, flake the tuna into small pieces with a fork. Add the carrot, celery, red and yellow pepper, scallion, mayonnaise, and lemon juice, and mix well with a fork.

Makes one serving

CHICKEN-APPLE SALAD CHOP

1 to 2 cups chopped romaine lettuce

4 ounces cooked chicken breast, shredded or chopped (canned or fresh)

¼ cup canned chickpeas (garbanzo beans), rinsed and drained

½ medium Fuji or McIntosh apple (with skin), chopped

¼ cup chopped cucumber (with peel)

¼ cup chopped tomato

¼ cup chopped celery

2 scallions, finely chopped

1 to 2 teaspoons olive oil with unlimited vinegar (or 2 tablespoons reduced-calorie vinaigrette)

Place the lettuce in a large bowl. Add the chicken, chickpeas, apple, cucumber, tomato, celery, and scallions. Drizzle with preferred dressing and gently toss to coat.

Makes one serving

WHOLE WHEAT PITA PIZZA

½ cup chopped broccoli florets

½ red bell pepper, thinly sliced

1 whole wheat pita bread, split (any brand 150 calories or less)

6 tablespoons marinara sauce

6 tablespoons (1½ ounces) shredded reduced-fat (part-skim) mozzarella cheese

Crushed red pepper flakes and oregano to taste

Sauté the broccoli florets and red pepper sticks in a pan coated with nonstick spray over medium heat until tender. (If preferred, broccoli and peppers may be softened in the microwave. Place in microwave-safe bowl with 2 tablespoons water and microwave on high for 2 to 3 minutes. Drain veggies before using.) Toast split pita bread. Top each pita half with 3 tablespoons marinara sauce and half the sautéed veggies. Sprinkle 3 tablespoons mozzarella cheese on each half. Heat in oven at 350°F until cheese melts and bubbles. Season with crushed red pepper and oregano.

Makes one serving

TURKEY TORTILLA ROLL UP

1 tablespoon reduced-fat mayo

Dijon mustard

1 whole wheat tortilla wrap (100 calories or less)

4 large lettuce leaves

4 ounces (¼ pound) sliced turkey breast or ham

4 slices red tomato

Pickles, onions, radishes, roasted peppers (optional)

Spread mayo and mustard on tortilla wrap.

Layer the lettuce, turkey, tomato, and vegetables. Now roll!

Makes one serving

STUFFED VEGETABLE OMELET

½ cup sliced mushrooms

½ cup diced onions

1 whole large egg and 3 egg whites

Preferred seasonings

Chopped tomato

In a pan sprayed with nonstick cooking spray, sauté the mushrooms and onions over medium heat until tender. Whip the egg and egg whites and pour over sautéed vegetables. Add the seasonings and continue to cook. When the bottom side is cooked, gently flip and cook the other side. Transfer to a plate and top with the tomato.

Makes one serving

OPEN-FACED TUNA MELT

1 can (6 ounces) chunk light tuna in water, drained (or chicken breast or wild salmon)

2 teaspoons reduced-fat mayonnaise

Minced onion, to taste

Preferred seasonings (including black pepper, dill, and mustard)

2 slices reduced calorie whole wheat bread (45 calories or less per slice)

½ thinly sliced tomato

Sliced onion and pickles (optional)

1 ounce reduced-fat or fat-free cheese, divided (any variety, including Swiss, cheddar, or American)

Drain and mash the tuna with mayonnaise, onion, and seasonings. Spread over bread that has been pre-toasted. Top each open slice with the tomato, onion, pickles, and cheese (½ ounce per slice). Place under the broiler or warm in an oven preheated to 350°F until cheese is hot and bubbly.

Makes one serving

OPEN-FACED TURKEY REUBEN

2 slices reduced calorie whole wheat bread, toasted

Sauerkraut

4 ounces turkey breast, divided

2 tablespoons reduced-fat Thousand Island (Russian) dressing*, divided

* You may use Joy's *LIFE* Thousand Island dressing (see recipe, page 61) or any brand 40 calories or less per 2 tablespoons

Toast the bread and top each slice with heaping spoonfuls of sauerkraut. Next layer each slice with 2 ounces of turkey breast. Spread Thousand Island dressing on top of turkey (1 tablespoon per slice).

Makes one serving

MINESTRONE SOUP

2 large onions, chopped

3 cloves garlic, minced (1 tablespoon)

4 slices low-fat turkey bacon, diced

4 ribs celery, chopped (about 2 cups)

5 carrots, sliced (about 2 cups)

2 cups (approximately 1 pound) fresh green beans, picked and cut into 1" pieces
   (may substitute frozen green beans)

8 cups lowfat chicken or vegetable broth (preferably low-sodium)

1 (28-ounce) can diced tomatoes (preferably low-salt)

1 (15-ounce) can kidney beans, drained

2 cups coarsely chopped baby spinach or arugula

4 cups diced zucchini

1 tablespoon dried oregano

1 tablespoon dried basil

3 bay leaves

Salt and pepper to taste

1. Spray a large stock pot with nonstick cooking spray and sauté onions and garlic over medium-low heat for 5 minutes. Add turkey bacon, celery, carrots, and green beans, and sauté for an additional 5 minutes.

2. Add the chicken broth and tomatoes; bring to a boil. Reduce heat to low and add the kidney beans, spinach or arugula leaves, zucchini, oregano, basil, and bay leaves. Simmer for 20 minutes, or until all vegetables are tender.

3. Season with salt and pepper to taste. Remove bay leaves before serving.

4. After being brought to room temperature, this soup can be frozen up to 2 months.

Makes 7 servings, 2 cups per serving

LIFE BLUEBERRY MANGO SMOOTHIE

½ cup cubed and frozen mango

½ cup blueberries, fresh or frozen, unsweetened

⅓ cup skim milk

2 tablespoons nonfat vanilla yogurt

3 ice cubes

Place first four ingredients in blender. Blend thoroughly, until smooth. Add ice cubes and puree until ice is crushed and drink is frosty.

Makes one serving

LIFE BANANA CARDAMOM SMOOTHIE

½ medium banana, sliced and frozen

½ cup nonfat vanilla yogurt

½ cup cold skim milk*

¼ teaspoon vanilla extract*

⅛ teaspoon ground cardamom

3 ice cubes

* May substitute ½ cup light vanilla soy milk in place of skim milk and vanilla extract.

Place first five ingredients in blender. Blend thoroughly, until smooth. Add ice cubes and puree until ice is crushed and drink is frosty.

Makes one serving

LIFE STRAWBERRY BANANA SMOOTHIE

1 full cup strawberries (about 7 whole medium)

½ medium banana

¾ cup cold skim milk

3 ice cubes

Place first three ingredients in blender. Blend thoroughly, until smooth. Add ice cubes and puree until ice is crushed and drink is frosty.

Makes one serving

LIFE CREAMSICLE SMOOTHIE

½ cup 100% orange juice

6 ounces nonfat, vanilla yogurt (any brand 100 calories or less per 6-ounce container)

3 to 5 ice cubes

Place orange juice and yogurt in blender. Blend thoroughly, until smooth. Add ice cubes and puree until ice is crushed and drink is frosty.

Makes one serving

SAVORY ALMONDS

1 egg white

2 teaspoons Old Bay seasoning

2 teaspoons Spanish paprika, sweet or hot

½ teaspoon cayenne pepper (optional)

2 teaspoons cumin powder, ground

1 teaspoon salt

1 tablespoon granulated sugar

1½ cups natural almonds

Preheat oven to 375°F. Prepare a nonstick baking sheet with cooking spray and set aside. In a large bowl, combine all the ingredients except the almonds. Add the almonds and stir to coat evenly. Place on the prepared baking sheet and bake for 15 minutes, stirring occasionally to evenly toast. Remove the almonds from the oven and allow to cool to room temperature. Store in an airtight container at room temperature for up to 1 week.

Makes approximately 9 servings, 20 almonds per serving

POPCORN SEASONING BLENDS

2 tablespoons unpopped popcorn kernels

Nonstick cooking spray, butter flavored

Makes one serving

Choose your seasoning blend:

Spanish "Tapas" Popcorn

½ teaspoon Spanish smoked paprika (mild or hot)

¼ teaspoon salt

Tex-Mex Popcorn

½ teaspoon chili powder

¼ teaspoon cumin

¼ teaspoon salt

Pinch of cayenne pepper (optional)

Parmesan-Black Pepper Popcorn

1 tablespoon finely grated Parmesan cheese

¼ teaspoon salt

¼ teaspoon fresh ground black pepper

Cinnamon Popcorn

½ teaspoon ground cinnamon

1 teaspoon confectioner's sugar

Pinch of salt

Put the popcorn kernels in a brown paper lunch bag and spray the kernels with nonstick cooking spray. Fold the bag over twice to seal. Shake the bag (while holding closed) to distribute nonstick spray evenly. Microwave on high about 2 minutes, or until popping slows to 2 seconds between pops. (Alternatively, you may use an air popper to make popcorn.) Pour the popped popcorn into a one gallon resealable bag. Liberally spray the popcorn with nonstick cooking spray and shake bag to distribute. Spray a second time with nonstick cooking spray and add preferred seasoning blend. SHAKE vigorously for 30 to 60 seconds . . . pour the contents into a bowl and enjoy!

GRAPEFRUIT ROSEMARY GRANITA

⅓ cup granulated sugar

⅔ cup water

2 to 3 fresh rosemary sprigs

2 cups pink grapefruit juice, freshly squeezed or bottled unsweetened

To create simple syrup, combine the sugar and water in a saucepan and bring to a simmer. Allow to simmer until the sugar has completely dissolved. Remove from heat and add the rosemary. Cover and allow to cool. (At this point the simple syrup can be placed in an airtight container and refrigerated for up to 2 weeks.) Remove the rosemary sprigs from the syrup and combine the syrup with grapefruit juice in 9 by 13-inch glass dish. Place in the freezer, check after 30 minutes, and lightly scrape the frozen areas with a fork. Continue to check and scrape every 20 to 30 minutes. When completely frozen, serve, or place in an airtight container in the freezer for up to 2 months.

If you would like a sorbet-type texture, place in a food processor when completely frozen. (No need to scrape with fork.) Process completely. Freeze in an airtight container for up to 2 months.

Makes 4 servings, ¾ cup each

BLUEBERRY MANGO SORBET

½ cup mango, cubed and frozen

½ cup blueberries, fresh or frozen, unsweetened

⅓ cup skim milk

2 tablespoons nonfat vanilla yogurt

3 ice cubes

Place all ingredients in a food processor. Process until smooth. Place in a small airtight bowl and freeze overnight.

Makes one serving

CREAMY VANILLA PUDDING

2½ cups plus ½ cup fat-free milk

¼ cup cornstarch

¼ cup sugar

1½ teaspoons vanilla extract

Heat 2½ cups milk to a simmer in a heavy-bottomed saucepan over medium heat. In a small bowl combine the sugar and cornstarch. Add the remaining ½ cup cold milk to the cornstarch and sugar mixture and whisk to combine, forming a slurry. Add the slurry to the simmering milk, whisking vigorously so the mixture does not scorch or clump. Continue cooking, stirring constantly, until the pudding is thick enough to coat the back of a spoon, about 2 to 3 minutes. Remove from the heat and stir in the vanilla. Pour into 4 dessert cups and refrigerate for at least two hours before serving.

Makes 4 servings, ¾ cup each

CREAMY CHOCOLATE PUDDING

2½ cups plus ½ cup fat-free milk

¼ cup sugar

¼ cup cornstarch

1 tablespoon unsweetened cocoa

1 teaspoon vanilla extract

Heat 2½ cups milk to a simmer in a heavy-bottomed saucepan over medium heat. In a small bowl combine the sugar, cornstarch, and cocoa. Add the remaining ½ cup cold milk to the cornstarch/sugar/cocoa mixture and whisk to combine, forming a slurry (make sure to break up any clumps of cocoa). Add the slurry to the simmering milk, whisking vigorously so the mixture does not scorch or clump. Continue cooking, stirring constantly, until the pudding is thick enough to coat the back of a spoon, about 2 to 3 minutes. Remove from the heat and stir in the vanilla. Pour into 4 dessert cups and refrigerate for at least two hours before serving.

Makes 4 servings, ¾ cup each

FUNKY MONKEY COFFEE DRINK

¾ cup cold coffee

½ peeled medium banana, sliced and frozen

1 tablespoon chocolate syrup

¼ cup nonfat vanilla yogurt

Place all the ingredients in a blender and blend thoroughly. Serve over ice cubes if desired.

Makes one serving

Recipes—Dinner and Sides

LIFE QUICHE

¼ cup diced onion

½ teaspoon dried basil

½ teaspoon dried oregano

½ cup chopped mushrooms

1 cup fresh spinach

Salt and pepper

2 large eggs

2 large egg whites

¼ cup skim milk

2 tablespoons fat-free half & half

1 medium tomato

1 ounce fat-free cream cheese

Preheat oven to 350°F. Coat small fry pan with cooking spray. Sauté the onion with basil and oregano over medium heat until soft, about 5 minutes. Add the mushrooms, spinach, salt and pepper to taste, and cook an additional 3 to 5 minutes or until soft. In a medium bowl, whisk together the eggs and egg whites, milk, and half & half. Slice four thin, round slices from the tomato; set the slices aside. Chop the remaining tomato into small cubes. Add the cooked vegetable mixture and chopped tomatoes to the beaten egg mixture. Coat a 9-inch pie dish with cooking spray and pour in the quiche mixture. Drop small pieces of cream cheese throughout the quiche mixture. Lay the tomato slices on top. Bake in 350°F oven for 30 to 40 minutes. Before removing from the oven, gently shake the pie dish; if the quiche is done, the center will appear firm.

Makes one serving

CHESAPEAKE SHRIMP BOIL

1 lemon (cut in half lengthwise)

3 garlic cloves, peeled and smashed

1 bay leaf

5 whole peppercorns

1 teaspoon salt

4 tablespoons Old Bay (or more to taste)

½ pound medium shell-on shrimp (approximately 15 to 18 shrimp)

Bring two quarts water to a boil. Squeeze the juice of both lemon halves into the water and toss the rinds into the pot. Add the garlic, bay leaf, peppercorns, salt, and seafood seasoning. Reduce the heat, and simmer, covered, for 15 minutes. Bring the water back to boil, add the shrimp and cook for 2 to 4 minutes (this will depend somewhat on the size of the shrimp). Remove the shrimp with slotted spoon into an individual bowl and spoon some of the cooking liquid over top.

Makes one serving

STEWED OKRA AND TOMATOES

2 tablespoons chopped onion

½ clove garlic, minced (½ teaspoon) (optional)

½ can (14½ ounces) diced tomatoes, preferably no salt added

1 cup cut okra, frozen or fresh

⅛ teaspoon red pepper flakes (optional)

Heat a small saucepan sprayed with nonstick cooking spray over medium heat. Add the onion and garlic and sauté until softened. Add the tomatoes, okra, and red pepper. Bring to a boil, then simmer, uncovered, over medium-low heat for 10 to 15 minutes, until most of the liquids have evaporated.

Makes one serving

EASY CHICKEN PUTTANESCA

5 ounce boneless skinless chicken breast, cut into 1" chunks

Salt and pepper

½ (14½-ounce) can diced tomatoes, preferably no salt added

6 kalamata olives, pitted and chopped (available at olive bar in grocery store)

½ cup artichoke hearts, coarsely chopped (frozen or canned in water, rinsed and drained)

Pinch crushed red pepper flakes

¼ teaspoon oregano

¼ teaspoon basil

⅛ teaspoon garlic powder

Sauté the chicken over medium high heat in a nonstick pan coated with cooking spray until browned and cooked through. Season with salt and pepper to taste. Add tomatoes, olives, artichoke hearts, and seasonings. Cover and simmer over medium low heat for 10 to 15 minutes.

Makes one serving

CHICKEN FLORENTINE

6 ounce boneless skinless chicken breast

Salt and pepper

1 garlic clove, minced

2 tablespoons minced shallot (1 medium)

½ teaspoon basil

½ teaspoon oregano

¼ cup low-sodium chicken stock

2 tablespoons skim milk

2 tablespoons fat-free half & half

1½ tablespoons plus ½ tablespoon grated Parmesan cheese

1 cup steamed spinach (frozen or fresh)

Preheat oven to 350°F. Cover 8-inch fry pan with cooking spray and heat over medium. Season the chicken breast with salt and pepper on both sides. Place the chicken breast in a pan and cook for approximately 5 minutes (until lightly browned); flip the chicken and cook for another 3 to 5 minutes. Remove from the pan and place on a small baking sheet. Place in preheated oven for approximately 8 to 10 minutes to finish cooking. With fry pan still on heat, spray with additional cooking spray, then add the garlic, shallot, basil, and oregano. Cook until soft, add the chicken stock, and reduce to 1 tablespoon (this will not take very long, so watch the pan). Add the milk, half & half, salt, and pepper. Let simmer for 5 to 7 minutes, take off heat and add 1½ tablespoons Parmesan cheese. Remove the chicken breast from the oven, slice across the grain to make 4 to 5 thick slices. On a serving plate, pour half of the Florentine sauce over the hot spinach. Place the sliced chicken breast atop, spoon the remaining sauce over, and top with the remaining ½ tablespoon Parmesan cheese.

Makes one serving

TANDOORI HALIBUT KEBABS

Tandoori Marinade:

⅓ cup fat-free plain yogurt or fat-free Greek yogurt

1½ teaspoons curry powder

¼ teaspoon turmeric powder

¼ teaspoon cayenne pepper

1 tablespoon honey

1½ teaspoons freshly grated ginger root (or ⅛ teaspoon ground ginger)

salt and pepper

Kebabs:

10 ounce halibut fillet, skin removed (or other firm white fish)

1 bell pepper (any color), seeded and cut into 1" chunks

1 small red onion, skin removed and cut into 1" chunks

½ cup grape or cherry tomatoes

Preheat the oven to 450°F. Prepare the Tandoori marinade: combine the yogurt, spices, honey, and grated ginger root in a medium bowl and mix thoroughly. Season marinade with salt and pepper to taste. Cut the halibut filet into 1" cubes and add to the marinade. Toss to coat. The fish may be marinated for up to 4 hours or may be used immediately. Thread the vegetables with the marinated halibut on 8" skewers, alternating fish with vegetables (approximately 3 halibut cubes per kebab). Place the kebabs an inch apart on a baking sheet lined with aluminum foil and sprayed with nonstick cooking spray (marinade will be sticky). Bake the skewers for 12 to 16 minutes, or until the halibut is firm to the touch.

Makes 2 servings, 3 kebabs per serving

PARMESAN BROILED TOMATO

½ large tomato, cut in half horizontally*

1 to 2 tablespoons Parmesan cheese

Pinch of garlic powder

Pinch of oregano

Salt and pepper

*Can substitute 1 small-medium tomato, with just top sliced off

Place the tomato on a small baking sheet sprayed with nonstick cooking spray or lined with aluminum foil. Spread the Parmesan over the cut side of the tomato and sprinkle with seasonings. Spray the top of the tomato with nonstick cooking spray. Broil 10″ from the heat for 5 minutes or until the tomato is hot and topping is browned. Serve immediately.

Makes one serving

SHRIMP CEVICHE WITH LIME

½ pound medium shrimp (approximately 15 to 18 shrimp), peeled and deveined

1 tablespoon salt

¾ cup lime juice (approximately 5 limes)

½ cup finely diced red onion

1 clove garlic, finely diced

½ to 1 teaspoon jalapeno pepper, finely diced

1 cup cucumber, diced

¼ cup chopped fresh cilantro (optional)

Place the shrimp in 2 quarts boiling water with the salt and cook for 1 to 2 minutes. Drain the shrimp and immediately place them in an ice water bath (this will stop them from cooking further). Remove the shrimp from the ice bath and cut them into 1″ pieces. Add the lime juice and place the shrimp in the refrigerator for at least 30 minutes, and up to 1 hour. Add the onion, garlic, and jalapeno to the shrimp. Refrigerate for another 30 minutes. Add the cucumber and cilantro, stir to combine, and serve.

Makes one serving

LIFE SHEPHERD'S PIE

1 large onion, diced (about 1½ cups)

½ cup diced celery (about 2 ribs)

1 medium red pepper, diced (about 1 cup)

2 carrots, diced (about 1 cup)

1 pound lean ground turkey (at least 90% lean)

2 tablespoons tomato paste (preferably low-sodium)

1 tablespoon Worcestershire sauce

1 teaspoon paprika

1 cup fat-free low-sodium beef broth

Salt and pepper

3 cups Cauliflower Mashed "Potatoes" (page 69)

½ cup (2 ounces) shredded reduced-fat cheddar cheese

Preheat the oven to 350°F. Coat an 8- to 10-cup ceramic or glass gratin dish or a 9 by 9 by 2-inch-square baking dish with nonstick cooking spray.

In a large skillet coated with nonstick spray, sauté the onion, celery, red pepper, and carrot over medium high heat until the onions are translucent and all the vegetables are softened, 6 to 8 minutes. Add the turkey, increase the heat to high, and cook, stirring, until the turkey is no longer pink, 5 to 7 minutes longer.

Stir in the tomato paste, Worcestershire sauce, paprika, garlic powder, and thyme. Cook, stirring, for 2 minutes. Add the broth and cook for 2 to 3 minutes, until the turkey is cooked through and a light sauce forms. Season to taste with salt and pepper. Spread into the prepared casserole dish.

Spread the prepared "Cauliflower Mash" over the meat mixture. Sprinkle with the cheese. Bake, uncovered, until the topping is browned around the edges, 30 to 35 minutes.

Makes 4 servings, approximately 2 cups each

TURKEY SAUSAGE WITH SAUTÉED PEPPERS AND ONIONS

1 medium red bell pepper, thinly sliced

1 medium green bell pepper, thinly sliced

½ medium onion, thinly sliced

1 3-ounce lean poultry sausage link (any brand 150 calories or less per link)

Heat a pan coated with nonstick cooking spray over medium heat. Add the peppers and onions and sauté for 8 to 10 minutes until soft and lightly browned. In a separate pan sprayed with nonstick cooking spray, sauté the sausage over medium heat until fully cooked through. Remove the sausage from the pan and slice into ¼ inch rounds. Add cut sausage to the pan with the cooked vegetables and sauté together for an additional 1 to 2 minutes over medium heat.

Makes one serving

ORANGE DIJON PORK TENDERLOIN

6 ounce pork tenderloin medallion

Salt and pepper

2 tablespoons 100% orange juice

2 teaspoons Dijon mustard

1 teaspoon honey

⅛ teaspoon garlic powder

Preheat the oven to 425°F. Season pork medallion with salt and pepper. Preheat a sauté pan coated with nonstick cooking spray over medium-high heat. Add pork and brown all sides (2 to 3 minutes per side). Transfer browned pork to ovenproof dish and roast for 15 minutes in oven to finish cooking (internal temperature should be 160°F). Meanwhile, prepare orange Dijon sauce. In the same sauté pan used to brown pork, whisk together orange juice, mustard, honey, and garlic powder and place over medium heat. Simmer until the sauce thickens and reduces by about a third, 2 to 4 minutes. Remove pork from oven and let rest 5 minutes. Slice pork across the grain, arrange on a plate, and drizzle with sauce before serving.

Makes one serving

4 WOMEN . . . ALMOST 400 POUNDS!

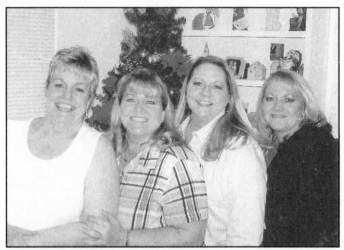

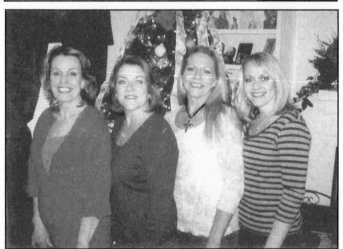

MARILYN MORRISON (mom)	SHERRY WHEATON	PENNY RUSSELL	ANNETTE HALBROOK
LOST: 118 pounds!	LOST: 65 pounds!	LOST: 95 pounds!	LOST: 115 pounds!
AGE: 64	AGE: 47	AGE: 44	AGE: 40
HEIGHT: 5'7"	HEIGHT: 5'4"	HEIGHT: 5'8"	HEIGHT: 5'6"
BEFORE: 255 pounds	BEFORE: 205 pounds	BEFORE: 235 pounds	BEFORE: 245 pounds
AFTER: 137 pounds	AFTER: 140 pounds	AFTER: 140 pounds	AFTER: 130 pounds

THIN ACCOMPLISHMENTS: Reviving the dreams of our younger days. We're a family who likes to give back. We've had a dream of opening an orphanage in Africa, but over the years, those dreams died. Now, we're starting to dig those old ideas up again. It feels like there are no limits!

THIN CHALLENGES: Food is emotional for us. As a family, we ate when we were happy, and we ate when we were sad. It has been a challenge to change that pattern.

WORDS OF WISDOM: When you peel away the fat, the real you is underneath. The things you want to do—the dreams you had when you were younger—you can finally do them.

HOW DID YOU ALL DECIDE TO LOSE WEIGHT TOGETHER?

Every year, we take a family picture. The "before" picture you see is from Christmas 2005. When this came back, Sherry sent a copy to everyone with a note that said, *See what we look like, ladies?* We were all appalled. Not only that, but we were all having health problems. That picture was enough to make us act.

DID IT HELP HAVING EVERYONE DIETING TOGETHER?

Definitely. We've always been a really close, loving family. We support each other and share everything. And we all wanted to get healthy together. Mom (Marilyn) has five great-grandchildren. We want her to be around to see her great-great-grandchildren.

ON CHANGING COOKING STYLES . . .

Down here in Texas, we fry anything that stands still. We even used to fry green beans! Now, our taste buds have changed. Healthy food just tastes better. Sherry says she can't even put fried food in her mouth anymore. It didn't take very long for that to happen.

CHANGE WHAT'S ON THE MENU. *In their heavier days, this family ate (and overate!) fried chicken, mashed potatoes with gravy, fried okra, butter-soaked corn on the cob, corn bread, and chocolate fudge cake topped with whipped cream. Now, their skinny menu includes grilled chicken, baked sweet potatoes, and sautéed asparagus and zucchini. Dessert is angel food cake with berries and reduced-fat whipped topping. The difference is more than 1,000 calories per plate!*

Step Three—*Reshape* 3

Welcome to the heart of Joy's LIFE Diet!

At this moment, you are on the verge of seeing dramatic changes in your body, your health, your energy levels . . . really, in all areas of your life. Can't you feel all that transformation potential bottled up inside you? It's there, trust me, otherwise you wouldn't have made it this far. Although I don't have any formal statistics, I know from experience that most people who successfully complete Steps One and Two will eventually reach their personal goal weight if they remain committed to that goal. You've done the hardest part. During those first three weeks, you stripped away the worst nutritional offenders and learned a new way of eating. In essence, you've pushed a great big reset button on your body's eating habits. The only things standing between you and your desired weight are dedication and time.

Step Three lasts as long as you need it to. This extended phase of Joy's LIFE Diet is your opportunity to *reshape* your body and reenergize your spirit. With each step closer to your goal, you may discover new facets of your personality that used to be hidden behind worries about being overweight. You may find new hobbies or activities that you never had the confidence to try before. One of the most moving stories I heard from a member of my Fit Club came from Mary Rosner, who, on her own, lost 180 pounds (read her profile on page 229). She and a friend decided to visit a lake that had no road access—the only way in was to hike over difficult and hilly terrain. At the end of a couple hours, they spied the lake, glorious and unspoiled. As she gazed out at this natural wonder, Mary cried. As she puts it, "I realized that if I hadn't lost the weight, I never would have seen it. It would have been physically impossible for me to hike that distance. I wept for the beauty of it, and for all the other wonders I probably already missed in my life. Now I want to see and do everything."

That's what Step Three is all about: helping you experience all those wonderful moments life has to offer. Just as with Mary's grueling lake expedition, the road may not always be easy, but it is definitely worth it!

Step Three Rules

In Step Three, you'll stick with the basic guidelines that were probably permanently embedded in your memory during Steps One and Two, but your hard work has also earned you several new freedoms. As always, feel free to repeat meals from Steps One and Two. And Step Three brings added flexibility. Because you have introduced starch with dinner, your dinners can be any breakfast or any lunch from any step. So if you would love to eat a bowl of cereal for dinner, or if you want to have a simple tuna melt, that's allowed in Step Three.

Here are some changes you can look forward to in Step Three:

1. *Portion-controlled starch with dinner.* In Step Three, starches make a comeback with dinner, which means you are sometimes allowed to enjoy old favorites like potatoes, rice, and pasta. Some dinners include starches and others, like those in Steps One and Two, do not. As usual, stick with the amounts specified in your meal plan.

2. *No pre-dinner soup/salad requirement.* In Steps One and Two, you started every evening meal with a *LIFE* Dinner Salad or bowl of *LIFE* Veggie Soup. In Step Three, this pre-dinner filler-upper is no longer mandatory. For those dinners in Step Three that do specify my *LIFE* soup or salad, you may choose to substitute one of the following items:

- **Shrimp cocktail:** Five shrimp with 1 heaping tablespoon ketchup mixed with 1 teaspoon horseradish, and/or unlimited optional fresh lemon.
- **Tomato and onion salad:** Sliced tomato and onion drizzled with plain balsamic vinegar or Joy's *LIFE* balsamic vinaigrette or 2 tablespoons of any reduced calorie vinaigrette (40 calories or less per 2 tablespoons)
- **HALF fruit serving:** Any HALF fruit serving, such as 1 orange, ½ banana, ¾ cup berries, or ½ cup chilled or frozen grapes

3. *150-calorie LIFE Extras.* In Step Two, you were given the option for one daily *LIFE* Healthy Extra (a fun food 150 calories or less). You were instructed to select your extra from an approved list of healthier snack options. In Step Three, you are now given the freedom to "spend" your 150 calories any way you choose. Because you may choose healthy foods or less-than-healthy foods, they are now simply called *LIFE* Extras. The only caveat is you must stay *at* or *below* the 150-calorie cutoff.

   You may continue to enjoy any of the healthier fun food options listed on pages 75–76—such as dark chocolate, frozen yogurt, or wine—or you may choose any of your personal favorite foods . . . anything goes! For instance, your 150 calories could buy you 4 cups of low-fat popcorn, 1 ounce of potato chips, 5 chocolate kisses, 2 forkfuls of your friend's decadent dessert, or 3 tablespoons of your grandma's secret recipe potato salad. You may also choose to double up on your designated portion of breakfast cereal, or include ½ of a medium baked potato (white or sweet), ½ cup of cooked pasta or rice with your dinner, or add one WHOLE fruit serving in the afternoon (each of these items provides about 120 calories). Of course, choosing less calorie-dense snacks will allow you to get more bang for your buck, but the choice is yours. You will be in charge of tracking the calories in your daily *LIFE* Extras. In fact, it's the only time you'll have to track calories on this plan, so make sure you pay close attention to the serving sizes listed on package nutrition labels. For help tracking your *LIFE* Extra calories, go to www.JoyBauer.com.

4. *Expanded Restaurant Guide with Fast-Food Options.* Joy's LIFE Diet is for real life, so I've included a larger list of restaurant options, including selections for fast-food aficionados.

OUTSMART FOOD LABELS!

When choosing 150-calorie *LIFE* Extras, you don't want to get hit with unexpected calories. The "Calories" line on a Nutrition Facts food label doesn't tell the full story.

The number of "Calories" really means "calories per serving," although that detail may not be immediately clear. The size of a serving is noted in the first line of the label (Serving Size). To understand how many total calories are in specific a can or package, look at the second line of the label (Servings Per Container) and multiply that number by the number listed next to "Calories." Use that number to guide your snack choices.

Step Three Food Rules: Dos and Don'ts

To summarize, here are the Dos and Don'ts for Step Three. Some of these rules will look familiar because you have been living with them for the past three weeks.

✗ 1. **DON'T** . . . add sugar to anything unless specified on the plan or in a recipe, or unless you count these calories as part of your *LIFE* Extra for the day.

✗ 2. **DON'T** . . . drink alcohol unless it's your *LIFE* Extra for the day.

✗ 3. **DON'T** . . . add salt to anything unless specified in a recipe.

✗ 4. **DON'T** . . . skip meals.

And . . .

✓ 5. **DO** . . . eat on a schedule and enjoy three meals and your afternoon snack each day.

✓ 6. **DO** . . . drink lots of water throughout the day, including two 8-ounce glasses *before* lunch and two 8-ounce glasses *before* dinner. (These before-meal waters should be consumed up to 30 minutes before eating.) Enjoy as much additional water as you want during meals and throughout the day.

✓ 7. **DO** . . . enjoy portion-controlled starches with some dinners (only when designated on your menu).

✓ 8. **DO** . . . take advantage of your option to begin dinner with *LIFE* Dinner Salad or *LIFE* Veggie Soup (see recipes on pages 59, 63), but only if you wish. These are optional in Step Three!

✓ 9. **DO** . . . feel free to enjoy one 150-calorie *LIFE* Extra each day at any time you like.

step three

BREAKFAST

+

LUNCH

▶ Two glasses water prior to eating your lunch

+

AFTERNOON SNACK

+

DINNER

▶ Two glasses of water prior to eating your dinner

SPECIAL NOTES

▶ Enjoy foods from Unlimited List any time throughout the day.

▶ All men and active women may eat unlimited protein portions at meals only.

▶ Enjoy one of *LIFE* Extras at any point during the day.

in a nutshell

✓10. **DO** . . . indulge in foods on the Unlimited Foods List (on pages 41–42). You can enjoy these foods in unlimited quantities at any time throughout the day, particularly when you get hungry between designated meal and snack times.

✓11. **DO** . . . feel free to swap meals or ingredients from within the same categories. Also, you may eat ANY breakfast for lunch, and ANY breakfast or lunch for dinner.

✓12. **DO** . . . enjoy meals listed in *LIFE* Restaurant Options when dining out (pages 56, 116)

✓13. **DO** . . . try different recipes for variety

✓14. **DO** . . . feel free to repeat a favorite meal or recipe during the week, as many times as you like (including menus from Step One and Step Two)

✓15. **DO** . . . feel free (if you choose) to consume up to two items each day with artificial sweetener, or no-calorie natural sweetener.

✓16. **DO** . . . feel free to substitute a frozen entrée for dinner on any night, as long as it's 350 calories or less

✓17. **DO** . . . follow Step Three exercise guidelines (page 272)

MELISSA LETTS

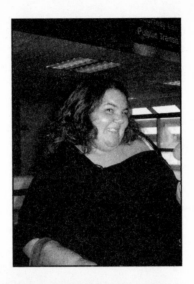

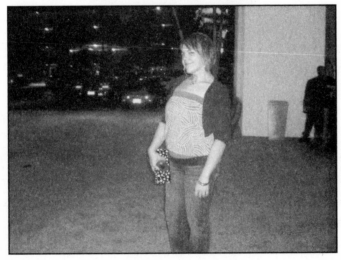

LOST: **165 pounds!**

AGE: **25**

HEIGHT: **5'4"**

BEFORE: **330 pounds, size 32**

AFTER: **165 pounds, size 10/12**

THIN ACCOMPLISHMENTS: I got my personal training certificate, and I work at a supplement store. I'm very health- and fitness-oriented right now. I'm trying to help people achieve goals I never thought I would have achieved for myself.

THIN CHALLENGES: I enjoy fitness, but sometimes it's tough when there are a million other things to do. As a trainer now, when my clients tell me they don't feel like working out, I can tell them, "I don't want to, either, so stop talking and keep moving."

WORDS OF WISDOM: Being thin is not a definition of what you are, it's a journey. It's a daily thing, and it's hard. But just because it's hard doesn't mean it's impossible. Just keep going.

WHAT WAS YOUR BIG WAKE-UP CALL?

I was in the operating room about to have gastric bypass surgery. Just as they were about to give me anesthesia, I stopped them, and told them to wheel me back. At the last minute, I feared having to give up food. I left, went to a Cracker Barrel restaurant, and stuffed my face. That's when I knew I had a problem.

WHAT DID YOU DO FROM THERE?

I started small so I wouldn't get overwhelmed. I aimed to lose just 10 pounds. I knew the overall goal, but I focused on the smaller goal. Every little thing I did gave results because I wasn't doing anything before! The big thing was that I didn't quit . . . before, I quit everything I started.

WHAT IS DIFFERENT ABOUT LIFE AFTER WEIGHT LOSS?

My life is 100 percent different. I tried to enroll in college, but I didn't fit in the desks so I never went back. I couldn't fit into restaurant booths so I didn't eat out. I didn't fit into movie theater seats. I didn't drive for years. Once I overcame my weight, I knew I could do anything.

The best was the other day when my son said to me, "I can hug you and fit my arms around you!"

JOY'S LESSONS LEARNED

MODIFY YOUR FAVORITE RECIPES. *Melissa grew up in Miami and has always loved traditional Cuban food. When she was inducted into my Joy Fit Club on TODAY, I taught her how to make lower calorie Cuban Picadillo (just 280 calories per cup!) and "Unfried" Plaintains. Anything can be prepared with less fat, sugar, and salt—you just have to be creative.*

Step Three Foods
Allowed At Meals
(Breakfast, Lunch, and Dinner)

This is the expanded list of foods incorporated into your 21-day Step Three meal plan. Like before, use this list to swap meats or other proteins specified in the meal plan for equivalent portions of any other meat or protein included on the Approved Foods list. For instance, if you'd rather forgo the roast beef in your *Classic Roast Beef Sandwich* on Day 13, you can substitute turkey, chicken breast, or lean ham. If you're getting tired of chicken, feel free to turn Day 14's *Sweet and Sour Chicken* into *Sweet and Sour Shrimp* instead.

As always, you can add or substitute any non-starchy vegetables in your meals and recipes. Be creative! Add fresh tomatoes to your *Fiesta Scrambled Eggs with Green Chiles* on Day 2, substitute carrots or zucchini in your side of *Balsamic Roasted Asparagus* on Day 18, or add some snow peas and/or water chestnuts to your *Teriyaki Vegetables* on Day 16.

Even though you have transitioned into Step Three, you can still continue to repeat breakfasts, lunches, dinners, and snacks from Step One and Step Two. That means you actually have six weeks worth of menus to work with . . . more than enough to keep the diet doldrums at bay! For example, if you would rather skip the *Crab Salad Plate* listed for lunch on Day 20 of Step Three, you have tons of replacement options. To name just a few, you could repeat the *Broccoli and Cheese Omelet* from Day 4 of Step One, repeat the *Open Faced Tuna Melt* from Day 8 of Step Two, or enjoy another lunch from Step Three (such as *LIFE Chef's Salad* from Day 11 or the *Vermont Turkey Sandwich* from Day 2). You are totally in control! (Items new to the foods allowed list are highlighted in **bold print**.)

Foods Allowed at Meals

*(Wallet-sized printable lists of allowed foods for each step are available at www. JoyBauer.com)

Meats

Lean cuts only:

+ Bottom round
+ Buffalo
+ Filet mignon
+ Flank
+ **Ground sirloin (at least 90% lean)**
+ London broil
+ **Lean deli roast beef**
+ Sirloin
+ Top round
+ Veal
+ Venison

Poultry (skinless only)

+ Chicken breast
+ Chicken breast, ground (at least 90% lean)
+ Chicken thigh
+ Cornish hen
+ Ostrich
+ Poultry sausage (lean)
+ Turkey bacon
+ Turkey breast
+ Turkey burger (lean)
+ Turkey thigh
+ Turkey, ground (at least 90% lean)

Pork

- **Canadian bacon**
- Ham, lean
- Pork tenderloin

Fish and seafood

- Anchovies
- Catfish
- Clams
- Cod
- Crab (fresh, canned, or imitation)
- Flounder
- Haddock
- Halibut
- Lobster
- Lox (smoked salmon)
- Mackerel (Atlantic only, not king)
- Mahi mahi
- Mussels
- Oysters
- Red snapper
- Salmon, wild (fresh, canned, and smoked)
- Sardines
- Scallops
- Shrimp
- Sole
- Tilapia
- Trout
- Tuna (canned light in water)
- Whitefish

Eggs

- ✦ Egg whites
- ✦ Egg substitute
- ✦ Eggs, whole (stick with noted amounts)

Vegan Proteins

- ✦ Soy milk (low-fat)
- ✦ Soy yogurt (nonfat and low-fat)
- ✦ Tempeh
- ✦ Tofu

BREAKFAST PROTEIN SUBSTITUTIONS

Within *LIFE* Diet Step Three menus, you can substitute equivalent amounts of different proteins. Sometimes the substitution is obvious (such as swapping 5 ounces chicken for 5 ounces salmon), but other times it can be difficult to know exactly what makes for a good substitution. Here are some of my favorite breakfast suggestions, along with appropriate portion conversions.

INSTEAD OF . . .	TRY THIS!
1 hard boiled egg	4 egg whites, hard boiled or scrambled -or-
	3 slices turkey bacon -or-
	½ cup fat-free or 1% low-fat cottage cheese -or-
	1 cup skim milk or plain nonfat yogurt -or-
	1 cup (8 oz) plain nonfat yogurt -or-
	6 ounce nonfat, flavored yogurt, any brand 100 calories or less

- ✦ Vegan cheese (nonfat and low-fat)
- ✦ Veggie burgers
- ✦ Wheat gluten/seitan

Dairy

- ✦ Cheese, fat-free (all varieties)
- ✦ Cheese, reduced-fat (all varieties)
- ✦ **Cheese, feta**
- ✦ **Cheese, gorgonzola**
- ✦ Cheese, Parmesan
- ✦ Cheese, Romano
- ✦ Greek yogurt (nonfat)
- ✦ Yogurt, nonfat plain and flavored (all brands 100 calories or less per 6-ounce container)

Vegetables (non-starchy only)

- ✦ Artichokes and artichoke hearts
- ✦ Asparagus
- ✦ Beans, non-starchy: green, yellow, Italian, and wax
- ✦ Beets
- ✦ Bok choy (Chinese cabbage)
- ✦ Broccoli
- ✦ Broccoli rabe
- ✦ Broccolini
- ✦ Brussels sprouts
- ✦ Cabbage
- ✦ Carrots
- ✦ Cauliflower
- ✦ Celery
- ✦ Dark green leafy vegetables:
  - ✦ Beet greens
  - ✦ Collard greens

- Dandelion greens
- Kale
- Mustard greens
- Spinach
- Swiss chard
- Turnip greens
- Eggplant
- Fennel
- Garlic
- Green onions (scallions)
- Jicama
- Leeks
- Lettuce:
  - Arugula
  - Endive
  - Escarole
  - Iceberg
  - Mixed greens/salad blends
  - Romaine
- Mixed vegetable blends without corn, starchy beans, peas, pasta, or any kind of sauce
- Mushrooms
- Okra
- Onion
- Peppers (all varieties)
- Pickles
- Pumpkin (fresh, frozen/canned—must say "100% pure pumpkin," no sugar added)
- Radicchio
- Radishes
- Rhubarb
- Red peppers (if packed in oil, pat dry)
- Sauerkraut

- Sea vegetables (nori, etc.)
- Shallot
- Snow peas
- Spaghetti squash
- Sprouts (all varieties)
- Summer (yellow) squash
- Tomato
- Water chestnuts
- Watercress
- Zucchini

Starchy Vegetables

Starchy vegetables are part of Step Three menus only within *specific* breakfast, lunch, and dinner recipes, and some afternoon snack options. You may also choose to eat them as your daily 150-calorie *LIFE* Extra—but be sure to check your portions carefully.

- Beans (legumes)
- **Corn**
- Green peas
- Lentils
- Sweet potato
- **White potato**

Whole Grains

Whole grains are incorporated into Step Three menus within specific breakfasts, lunches, snacks, and dinners. Eat whole grain items only when designated at a particular meal, or choose to eat them as your daily 150-calorie *LIFE* Extra—but be sure to check your portions carefully.

- **Joy Bauer *LIFE* Bars**
- *LIFE* Muffins (see recipes pages 119–123)

- ✦ Mini whole wheat pita bread (no more than 70 calories)
- ✦ Regular whole wheat pita bread (no more than 150 calories)
- ✦ Reduced calorie whole wheat bread (no more than 45 calories per slice)
- ✦ Rice cakes (stick with plain, 45 calories per rice cake)
- ✦ Wheat germ
- ✦ Whole grain bread (any brand that lists "whole wheat" as first ingredient)
- ✦ Whole grain cereal (any brand 120 calories or less per ¾ to 1 cup serving; no more than 6 grams sugar; at least 3 grams fiber)
- ✦ Whole grain English muffin (any brand 130 calories or less)
- ✦ Whole grain oats (plain flavor only; traditional, quick cooking, or steel cut oats)
- ✦ Whole grain tortilla wrap (no more than 100 calories per wrap)
- ✦ Whole grain waffles (no more than 170 calories per two waffles)
- ✦ **Whole wheat pasta**
- ✦ **Brown rice**
- ✦ **Whole wheat couscous**
- ✦ **Hotdog buns (preferably whole grain)**
- ✦ **Bread crumbs (preferably whole grain)**
- ✦ **Taco shells (soft or hard)**

Fruit

Fruit is incorporated into Step Three menus within specific breakfast, lunch, and dinner recipes, and some afternoon snack options. Eat fruit only when designated for a particular meal. Make careful note to eat only the amount listed—some meals list "HALF servings" and others list "WHOLE servings." (Note: When making substitutions, be sure to pick from the right serving size.)

HALF Fruit Serving Options
- ✦ Apple: 1 small (palm-sized)
- ✦ Apricot: 6 dried halves, or 3 whole (fresh or dried)
- ✦ Banana: ½ medium

- ✦ Berries: ¾ cup (fresh or frozen, unsweetened blueberries, raspberries, black-berries, boysenberries, or sliced strawberries; or 10 whole strawberries)
- ✦ Cantaloupe: ¼ medium or 1 cup cubed
- ✦ Cherries (fresh): ½ cup (about 10 whole)
- ✦ Clementines: 2
- ✦ Fruit salad: ½ cup fresh cut (from produce section, unsweetened)
- ✦ Grapefruit: ½ (red, pink, or white)
- ✦ Grapes (seedless): ½ cup (red, purple, green, or black)
- ✦ Honeydew melon: 1 cup cubed
- ✦ Kiwi: 1 whole
- ✦ Mango: ½ fresh or ½ cup chunks (unsweetened)
- ✦ Nectarine: 1 whole
- ✦ Orange: 1 medium
- ✦ Papaya (fresh): 1 cup cubed
- ✦ Peach: 1 whole
- ✦ Pear: ½ large or 1 small
- ✦ Plum: 1 large
- ✦ Pomegranate: ½ medium
- ✦ Prunes: 3
- ✦ Raisins: 2 tablespoons
- ✦ Tangerine: 1 whole
- ✦ Watermelon, 1 cup cubed

WHOLE Fruit Serving Options

- ✦ Apple: 1 large
- ✦ Apricot: 12 dried halves, or 6 whole (fresh or dried)
- ✦ Banana: 1 whole
- ✦ Berries: 1½ cups (fresh or frozen, unsweetened blueberries, raspberries, blackberries, boysenberries, or sliced strawberries; or 20 whole strawberries)
- ✦ Cantaloupe: ½ medium or 2 cups cubed
- ✦ Cherries (fresh): 1 cup (about 20 whole)
- ✦ Clementines: 3
- ✦ Fruit salad: 1 cup fresh cut (from the produce section, unsweetened)

- Grapefruit: 1 whole (red, pink, or white)
- Grapes (seedless): 1 cup (red, purple, green, or black)
- Honeydew melon: 2 cups cubed
- Kiwi: 2 large
- Mango: 1 medium fresh or 1 cup chunks (unsweetened)
- Nectarines: 2
- Oranges: 2 medium
- Papaya (fresh): 2 cups cubed
- Peaches: 2 large
- Pear: 1 large
- Pineapple chunks: 1 cup fresh
- Plums: 2 large
- Pomegranate: 1 medium
- Prunes: 6
- Raisins: ¼ cup
- Tangerines: 2
- Watermelon: 2 cups cubed

Seasonings, Condiments, Marinades, and Healthy Fats

Your meal plans for Step Three make use of the following ingredients to flavor and jazz up your meals. Some of the condiments, such as vinegar, mustard, and hot sauce, are also included on the Unlimited List (see pages 35–36) and therefore can be added in unlimited quantities to ANY meal or snack, whether specified or not. For items not found on the Unlimited List, such as ketchup, mayo, and salad dressings, always stick with the portions designated in your meal plan.

- Avocado
- **Barbecue sauce** (any brand, 40 calories or less per 2 tablespoons)
- **Capers**
- Chiles or hot peppers, fresh or canned in vinegar/water
- **Chili sauce**
- Extracts (vanilla, almond, peppermint, etc.)

- Fruit jam
- Honey
- Horseradish
- Hot sauce
- Ketchup
- Lemon, fresh
- Lime, fresh
- Maple syrup (real or reduced calorie/sugar)
- Marinara sauce (opt for brands with 60 calories or less per half-cup serving)
- Mayo, reduced-fat (any brand, 25 calories or less per tablespoon)
- Mustard (plain, brown, spicy, Dijon)
- Nonstick cooking spray (any variety)
- Nuts (almonds, pistachios, walnuts, etc.)
- Nut butters (peanut, soy, almond, etc.)
- Olive oil
- Olives
- Orange juice, 100% fruit
- Salad dressing, Caesar (only use for Caesar salad lunch option—any brand, no more than 80 calories per 2 tablespoons)
- Salad dressing, low-calorie (any brand with no more than 40 calories per 2 tablespoons)
- Salad dressing, Joy's *LIFE* recipes (pages 60–63)
- Salsa (mild or spicy; any brand without added sugar or corn syrup)
- Salt substitute
- **Sesame seeds**
- Soy sauce, low-sodium
- Steak sauce
- Sugar, brown or white
- Teriyaki sauce, low-sodium
- **Tomato juice**
- Vinegar, any type—not vinaigrette
- Wasabi

- ✦ Worcestershire sauce
- ✦ Herbs and Spices
  - ✦ Allspice
  - ✦ Anise seed
  - ✦ Basil
  - ✦ Bay leaves
  - ✦ Cardamom
  - ✦ Cayenne pepper
  - ✦ Celery seed
  - ✦ Chili powder
  - ✦ Chinese five-spice
  - ✦ Chives
  - ✦ Cilantro
  - ✦ Cinnamon
  - ✦ Cloves
  - ✦ Coriander
  - ✦ Cumin
  - ✦ Curry powder
  - ✦ Dill weed
  - ✦ Garlic powder
  - ✦ Ginger
  - ✦ Lemongrass
  - ✦ Marjoram
  - ✦ Mint
  - ✦ Mustard
  - ✦ Mustard seed
  - ✦ Nutmeg
  - ✦ Old Bay seasoning
  - ✦ Onion powder
  - ✦ Oregano
  - ✦ Paprika
  - ✦ Parsley

- ✦ Pepper (ground) and whole peppercorns
- ✦ Pumpkin pie spice
- ✦ Red pepper flakes
- ✦ Rosemary
- ✦ Sage
- ✦ Seasoning blends
- ✦ Tarragon
- ✦ Thyme
- ✦ Turmeric

Beverages

- ✦ Club soda
- ✦ Coffee (no added sugar, no artificial sweeteners unless counted toward your daily allotment, no cream or whole milk. You may add skim, 1% or low-fat soy milk only.)
- ✦ Naturally flavored zero-calorie coffee with no artificial sweeteners (see recipes page 37)
- ✦ Diet soda and other artificially sweetened beverages (each 12-ounce can or 20-ounce bottle counts as half of your daily artificial sweetener allotment)
- ✦ Seltzer, zero calorie (plain and naturally flavored)
- ✦ Sparkling water
- ✦ Tea (black, white, green, herbal—no added sugar or honey; no added artificial sweeteners unless counted toward your daily allotment)
- ✦ Water
- ✦ Naturally flavored waters, calorie-free (see recipes page 38)

ACCEPTABLE MID-AFTERNOON SNACKS (100 to 150 calories)

You may substitute afternoon snacks listed on your menu with the following options. Stick with one per day, and pay close attention to designated portions.

Cheese Options

- 1 ounce reduced-fat or fat-free cheese with unlimited celery and pepper sticks
- 1 ounce reduced-fat or fat-free cheese with 1 mini whole-grain pita (no more than 70 calories) or rice cake
- 1 ounce reduced-fat or fat-free cheese with 10 raw almonds or 15 pistachio nuts
- 1 part-skim cheese stick with a HALF fruit serving (see list)
- 4 level tablespoons reduced-fat cream cheese with unlimited celery sticks
- ½ cup low-fat or nonfat cottage cheese, topped with a HALF fruit serving
- ½ cup low-fat or nonfat cottage cheese with unlimited non-starchy vegetables (i.e., cherry tomatoes, red pepper strips, celery, or baby carrots)
- ¾ cup low-fat or nonfat cottage cheese, plain or with cinnamon
- 1 slice reduced calorie, whole-grain toast (any brand 45 calories or less per slice) with 1 ounce slice reduced or nonfat cheese and optional tomato slices
- 1 slice reduced calorie, whole-grain toast (any brand, 45 calories or less per slice) with 1 level tablespoon reduced-fat cream cheese
- **½ cup low-fat or nonfat cottage cheese mixed with ½ cup canned crushed pineapple (canned in its own juice and drained)**
- **1 dry toasted whole-grain English muffin (any brand, 130 calories or less) topped with 2 teaspoons fat-free cream cheese**

Yogurt Options

- 8 ounces nonfat plain, Greek, or any flavored yogurt (150 calories or less)
- 6 ounces nonfat plain, Greek, or any flavored yogurt (100 calories or less), topped with 2 tablespoons wheat germ or ground flaxseed
- 6 ounces nonfat plain, Greek, or any flavored yogurt (100 calories or less), topped with a HALF fruit serving
- Vanilla Pumpkin Pudding: 6 ounces nonfat vanilla yogurt (any brand, 100 calories or less) mixed with ½ cup 100% pure pumpkin puree and cinnamon to taste
- **Bananas and Cream: 6 ounces nonfat vanilla yogurt (any brand, 100 calories or less) mixed with ½ banana, thinly sliced**

Nut and Nut Butter Options

- 10 raw almonds or 15 pistachios and a HALF fruit serving
- 10 raw almonds or 15 pistachios and ½ cup (one snack container) no-sugar-added natural applesauce
- 20 raw almonds
- 30 pistachios
- 2 level teaspoons natural peanut butter and a HALF fruit serving, i.e., ½ banana or 1 small apple
- 1 level tablespoon natural peanut butter with unlimited celery sticks
- 1 slice reduced calorie, whole-grain toast (any brand, 45 calories or less per slice) with 1 level tablespoon natural peanut butter
- **2 rice cakes (any brand, 45 calories or less per cake) + one teaspoon peanut, almond, apple, or soy nut butter**

Fruit Options

- 1 frozen banana
- 1 cup frozen grapes
- One WHOLE fruit serving
- 1 orange (or any other HALF fruit serving) and 1 mini whole-grain pita (no more than 70 calories)
- 1 *LIFE* Smoothie (see recipe pages 132–133)
- **Banana Split: 1 banana, split lengthwise and topped with 2 tablespoons reduced-fat whipped topping**
- **12-ounce skim latte or cappuccino with optional 1 teaspoon/packet sugar or artificial sweetener + small apple (or any HALF fruit serving)**

Vegetable Options

- **Half a medium baked potato (sweet or white) topped with 2 tablespoons salsa, ketchup, or nonfat sour cream**
- **1 regular whole wheat pita (or 2 mini pitas), cut into wedges, sprayed with nonstick cooking spray and baked at 375°F for 10 to 15 minutes + 2 tablespoons salsa**

- ✦ Curry Sweet Potato Fries (see recipe page 220)
- ✦ 2 cups *LIFE* soup with 1 mini whole wheat pita (any brand, 70 calories or less per pita) *or* 1 slice reduced calorie whole wheat toast (any brand, 45 calories or less per slice) *or* 60 to 70 calories worth of whole grain crackers
- ✦ Spinach or Broccoli Marinara: Microwave one 10-ounce package frozen chopped spinach or broccoli until cooked. Thoroughly drain and mix with 2 heaping tablespoons marinara sauce. Place back in microwave and reheat for 45 seconds. Top with optional 2 tablespoons Parmesan or reduced-fat shredded cheese.

Miscellaneous Options

- ✦ 4 ounces turkey breast rolled with lettuce and mustard
- ✦ 1 mini whole-grain pita (no more than 70 calories) with 2 level tablespoons hummus (any variety)
- ✦ ¼ cup hummus (any variety) with unlimited cucumber slices, celery sticks, and/or red, yellow, and green bell pepper strips
- ✦ 1 cup edamame beans boiled in the pod (green soybeans, fresh or frozen)
- ✦ ½ medium ripe avocado drizzled with lime juice, salt and pepper to taste
- ✦ 1 rice cake + one hard boiled egg (or 4 egg whites)
- ✦ 1 slice reduced calorie whole-grain toast (any brand, 45 calories or less per slice) topped with one hard boiled egg mashed and mixed with minced onion and 1 teaspoon reduced-fat mayonnaise.
- ✦ 1 *LIFE* Muffin (see recipe pages 119–123)
- ✦ 1 Joy Bauer *LIFE* Bar
- ✦ **Hummus Deviled Eggs: 2 hard boiled eggs, halved lengthwise and yolks replaced with a total of ¼ cup hummus (any variety)**
- ✦ **150 calories worth of soy crisps (any flavor variety)**
- ✦ **4 cups low-fat popcorn (any prepared or microwaveable brand 30 calories or less per cup, with or without low-calorie *LIFE* seasoning blends. See recipe for homemade varieties, page 134)**

UNLIMITED FOOD/BEVERAGE LIST

Enjoy in unlimited amounts—at any time of the day.

- ✦ ALL non-starchy vegetables! (see vegetables list on pages 295–296)
- ✦ Club soda (with optional fresh lemon or lime)
- ✦ Coffee (black, or with skim, 1% or soy milk only; no sugar)
- ✦ Naturally flavored zero-calorie coffee with no sugar (see recipes page 37)
- ✦ Extracts (vanilla, almond, peppermint, etc.)
- ✦ Herbs and spices (see list on pages 35–36)
- ✦ Horseradish
- ✦ Hot sauce
- ✦ Lemon and lime wedges
- ✦ Low-sodium broth
- ✦ Mustard (plain, brown, spicy, Dijon)
- ✦ Nonstick cooking spray (any variety)
- ✦ Joy's *LIFE* Balsamic Vinaigrette Salad Dressing
- ✦ Salsa (mild or spicy; any brand without added sugar or corn syrup)
- ✦ Salt substitute
- ✦ Seltzer water (plain or naturally flavored with optional fresh lemon or lime)
- ✦ Sparkling water
- ✦ Soy sauce, low-sodium
- ✦ **Sugar-free gum**
- ✦ Tea (iced or hot, with lemon *or* skim, 1% or soy milk only; no sugar or honey)
- ✦ Vinegar (any variety)
- ✦ Wasabi
- ✦ Water (with optional fresh lemon or lime)
- ✦ Naturally flavored waters, calorie-free (see recipes page 38)
- ✦ Worcestershire sauce

PATTI CARLSON

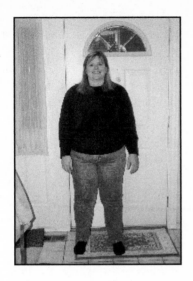 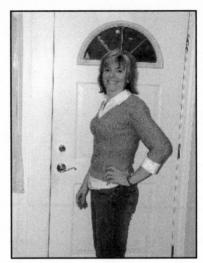

LOST: **125 pounds!**

AGE: **45**

HEIGHT: **5'5"**

BEFORE: **270 pounds, size 22**

AFTER: **145 pounds, size 6/8**

THIN ACCOMPLISHMENTS: In training for a sprint triathlon. It is a half-mile swim, a 13.8-mile bike ride, and a 3.1-mile run. I didn't know how to swim, so I took a triathlon training class. It took everything I had mentally to go back the second week of class, but I went. I learned a lot.

THIN CHALLENGES: Once I start eating certain foods, I cannot stop. Now I have certain boundaries with food I cannot cross over. For example, I cannot have Ben & Jerry's ice cream ever again. Or bakery doughnuts. Or a Hostess cherry pie. Now I don't buy them; they're never in the house.

WORDS OF WISDOM: The concept of "cheating" on a diet makes no sense. If you cheat, you're only cheating yourself.

WHAT STARTED YOU ON THE ROAD TO WEIGHT LOSS?

I knew I wanted to lose weight, but I didn't think I could do it on my own. I interviewed to be on a weight loss reality show, but I didn't get called back. I got angry, and said, "The heck with them. I can do this on my own." The next morning, I got on the treadmill for 15 minutes, and I pretended I had a trainer telling me to keep moving. There was no stopping me after that.

IT WAS THAT EASY?

I had this tremendous determination. It was like having an on/off switch in my head. It flipped, I was done—done being overweight, done being tired all the time, done with it all. I didn't want to be that person anymore. I was going to remake myself.

ON FINDING THE RIGHT TIME TO START EATING BETTER . . .

I started on December 12. My friends said, "Why not wait until after Christmas?" I planned to do this for the rest of my life, so it didn't matter when I started.

ON BATTLING STRESS EATING . . .

I have a lot of vacation days saved up, but I'm a little afraid to take them because the structure of work keeps me in line. Instead of vacationing, I exercise. I go to a 5:30 am spinning class. By the end of the class, I feel wonderful. It is an unbelievable stress reducer, my time for sanity.

JOY'S LESSONS LEARNED

THE RIGHT TIME TO START LOSING WEIGHT IS . . . *NOW! Don't wait until Monday . . . or next month . . . or after your birthday . . . or any other arbitrary start date. It's all just procrastination. START RIGHT THIS MINUTE!*

Step Three
Menus and Recipes

On the following pages are meal plans for the full 21 days of Step Three. Feel free to repeat or swap corresponding meals—breakfast for breakfast, lunch for lunch, or dinner for dinner (from among Steps One, Two, and Three meals). Any breakfast meal may now also be enjoyed for lunch or dinner, and any lunch may now be enjoyed at dinner. If you're a member of the online program at www.JoyBauer.com, you'll be able to browse even more Step Three meals and recipes.

For a list of the easiest, low-prep meals for Step Three, see pages 200–201.

In the event that you eat out, follow my LIFE Diet Step Three Restaurant Options on page 202.

Special Instructions for All Men and Some Active Women

(Follow these instructions if you are a man, or if you are a woman under age 40 who does more than one hour of cardiovascular exercise at least six days each week.) Although specific portions are listed for protein at each meal (egg whites, meat, chicken, turkey, fish and seafood, and tofu), all men and active women may eat *unlimited* protein portions at meals only—that means breakfast, lunch, and dinner, but not with your snack or throughout the rest of the day.

Special Instructions for Vegetarians

Substitute low-fat soy milk, soy yogurt, and soy cheese for dairy products. For meat and poultry, substitute an equivalent portion of fish, seafood, tempeh, or meat analog products. If opting to replace meat with tofu, double the portion size listed (since tofu is less dense than meat). You may also substitute veggie burgers for turkey burgers or other meat entrées.

LIFE Extra

Enjoy an extra 150 calories each day.

Anything goes—you may choose any food or foods within the calorie limit.

BREAKFAST

Bananas and Cream

1 banana, thinly sliced and mixed with 6 ounces nonfat vanilla yogurt (any brand 100 calories or less) and 1 heaping tablespoon reduced-fat or nonfat sour cream (sprinkle with optional cinnamon).

LUNCH

Egg White Salad with English Muffin

Egg White Salad (page 282) with one dry toasted English muffin (any brand 130 calories or less)

Enjoy with unlimited celery sticks, baby carrots, and pepper strips.

SNACK

One WHOLE fruit serving

DINNER

Orange Dijon Pork Tenderloin (page 144)
Green Beans with Tangy Vinaigrette

Add 1 to 2 cups washed and trimmed green beans to microwave-safe dish with 3 tablespoons water.

Cover and microwave until tender-crisp, about 3 to 4 minutes. Drain.

In small bowl, whisk together 1 tablespoon red wine vinegar, ½ teaspoon olive oil, 1 teaspoon Dijon mustard, and salt and pepper to taste.

Microwave dressing for 10 to 15 seconds or until warm and drizzle over green beans.

BREAKFAST

Fiesta Scrambled Eggs with Green Chiles (page 213)

LUNCH

Vermont Turkey Sandwich

> Spread 1 to 2 teaspoons Dijon mustard onto 2 slices reduced calorie whole wheat bread.
>
> Top with 3 ounces turkey breast (or lean ham), 1 ounce reduced-fat cheddar cheese, and 3 slices apple (such as Granny Smith).
>
> Enjoy with rest of apple, sliced, alongside.

SNACK

Joy Bauer *LIFE* Bar

DINNER

Baked Fish

> Preheat oven to 400°F and prepare baking sheet with nonstick cooking spray.
>
> Place one (6 to 8 ounce) wild salmon or halibut fillet on baking sheet and season with lemon juice, salt, pepper, and other preferred seasonings.
>
> Roast for 15 to 20 minutes, or until fish is opaque and cooked through.

Sautéed Spinach (page 65)

BREAKFAST

Ricotta and Ham Toast

Lightly toast 2 slices reduced calorie whole wheat bread.

Top each slice with 2 level tablespoons low-fat (part-skim) ricotta cheese and 1 ounce lean ham or Canadian bacon. Season with black pepper. Place under broiler until hot.

LUNCH

Greek Salad with Feta (page 217)

SNACK

150 calories worth of soy crisps

DINNER

Barbecue Chicken

Grill or pan sauté in nonstick cooking spray one (6 ounce) boneless skinless chicken breast.

During last five minutes of cooking, coat with 1 to 2 tablespoons barbecue sauce.

Creamy Coleslaw for One (page 218)
Steamed Veggies

Enjoy unlimited steamed broccoli, cauliflower, Brussels sprouts, or sugar snap peas.

BREAKFAST

LIFE Bar with Yogurt

> *One Joy Bauer LIFE bar with 6 ounces nonfat plain, Greek, or flavored yogurt (any brand 100 calories or less—or any other breakfast protein).*

LUNCH

Ham and Cheese Sandwich

> *Two slices reduced calorie whole wheat bread with 3 ounces lean ham, 1 ounce reduced-fat cheese (any variety), and optional mustard or 1 tablespoon reduced-fat mayo.*
>
> *Enjoy with sliced cucumber or any other non-starchy vegetable.*

SNACK

> *HALF fruit serving+ 15 pistachios or 10 almonds.*

DINNER

Grilled Sirloin Steak

> *5 ounces lean steak, seasoned as desired with allowed marinades/herbs/seasonings.*
>
> *Preheat a large skillet or grill to medium-high heat and cook to preferred temperature.*
>
> *Enjoy with optional 2 tablespoons steak sauce, ketchup, or barbecue sauce.*

Tomato and Mozzarella Salad

> *Slice ½ medium tomato and 1 ounce reduced-fat (part-skim) mozzarella cheese.*
>
> *Line alternate slices of tomato and mozzarella on plate.*
>
> *Drizzle with 2 tablespoons LIFE balsamic vinaigrette (or other reduced calorie vinaigrette dressing).*

BREAKFAST

Fruit, Cheese, and Nuts "To Go"

1 part-skim mozzarella (or any reduced-fat) cheese stick

Any HALF fruit serving

15 natural whole almonds

LUNCH

Turkey Sausage with Sauerkraut and Mustard

One lean poultry sausage served on one standard hotdog bun, preferably whole grain, topped with unlimited sauerkraut and mustard.

Enjoy with crunchy celery sticks, pepper strips, and/or carrots.

SNACK

*Unlimited celery sticks with 4 rounded tablespoons fat-free cream cheese (**or** 2 rounded tablespoons reduced-fat cream cheese, **or** 1 level tablespoon peanut butter)*

DINNER

Crispy Oven Fried Cod (page 219)
Sweet Potato Fries (page 220)

Prepared with or without curry powder (may substitute ½ medium baked potato, sweet or white)

Steamed Green Beans

Unlimited

BREAKFAST

Vanilla French Toast (page 213)

Topped with ¾ cup berries (thawed from frozen or fresh), or any other HALF fruit serving.

(For simple fruit topping, mash berries or other fruit with fork and microwave 30 to 60 seconds to warm.)

LUNCH

Steamed Chinese Food

Order "steamed" chicken, shrimp, or tofu with vegetables. Request garlic sauce on the side and drizzle ONLY one tablespoon on your steamed entrée (you may add additional low-sodium soy sauce).

Avoid all extras including rice, dumplings, etc.

SNACK

*One **WHOLE** fruit serving*

DINNER

LIFE Dinner Salad (page 59)
Uncle Onion's Turkey Bean Chili (page 222)

1½ cups chili topped with 1 ounce shredded reduced-fat cheddar cheese and 1 tablespoon reduced-fat or nonfat sour cream.

BREAKFAST

Spinach and Feta Egg Scramble (page 214)

LUNCH

Minestrone Soup and Salad

> *2 cups minestrone, lentil, or black bean soup.**

> *Mixed green salad with 2 tablespoons light dressing **or** 1 teaspoon olive oil and unlimited vinegar and fresh lemon.*

> ** For store-bought soup, use any brand 300 calories or less per 2 cups.*

> *You may also choose to prepare **LIFE** Minestrone Soup (page 131). Or, add ¾ cup beans to **LIFE** Veggie Soup (pages 63–64).*

SNACK

> *One part-skim stick cheese+one orange or half grapefruit (or any HALF fruit serving).*

DINNER

Fish Fillet en Papillote with Garden Vegetables (page 223)

> *Served over ½ cup cannellini beans (or any other variety of beans).*

BREAKFAST

Open-Faced Toasted Tomato and Cheese Sandwich

2 slices reduced calorie whole wheat bread, toasted and topped with sliced tomato and 2 slices (¾ ounce each) reduced-fat cheese.

Place in oven or under broiler until cheese melts.

LUNCH

Heavy-on-the-Veggies Tuna Pasta Salad

Mix together one level ½ cup cooked whole wheat pasta (any short cut, such as penne or rotini) with one cup chopped non-starchy vegetables (celery, carrot, tomato, onion, bell pepper, cucumber, etc.) and one (6 ounce) can chunk light tuna in water, drained (or substitute with wild salmon or chicken breast).

Toss with 3 to 4 tablespoons reduced calorie vinaigrette or 1 teaspoon olive oil, unlimited vinegar, and desired herbs and seasonings.

SNACK

One WHOLE fruit serving.

DINNER

Italian Chicken

In resealable storage bag, add one (6 ounce) boneless, skinless chicken breast and 2 tablespoons reduced calorie Italian dressing (or 1 teaspoon olive oil, unlimited vinegar, and desired seasonings).

Seal bag and make sure chicken is completely coated. Marinate at least one hour, or overnight.

Grill, pan sauté, broil, or roast at 350°F for 25 to 30 minutes, or until chicken is cooked through.

Stuffed Portobello Mushroom Caps (page 227)

BREAKFAST

Yogurt with Fresh Fruit and Wheat Germ

One WHOLE fruit serving (such as ½ medium cantaloupe, one pear, or one whole grapefruit).

6 ounces nonfat plain, Greek, or flavored yogurt (any brand 100 calories or less).

2 tablespoons wheat germ.

LUNCH

LIFE Scallion Pancake with Sour Cream (page 218)

SNACK

Broccoli Marinara

Microwave one 10-ounce package of frozen chopped broccoli until cooked. Thoroughly drain and mix with 2 heaping tablespoons marinara sauce. Place back in microwave and reheat for 45 seconds. Top with optional 2 table-spoons grated Parmesan or reduced-fat shredded cheese.

DINNER

Steak Balsamica

Marinate 5 ounces lean steak in a resealable storage bag with 2 tablespoons balsamic vinegar, 1 clove (1 teaspoon) minced garlic (or ¼ teaspoon garlic powder), and black pepper for 30 minutes. Grill, pan sauté, or broil, cooking to preferred temperature.

Oven Roasted Parmesan Cauliflower

Preheat oven to 425°F. Spray baking sheet with nonstick cooking spray.

Add 2 to 3 cups raw cauliflower florets, spray tops with cooking spray, and sprinkle with 1 tablespoon Parmesan cheese, ⅛ teaspoon garlic powder, and salt and pepper to taste.

Roast 20 to 30 minutes, or until tops of cauliflower are brown and crispy.

BREAKFAST

Cereal with Milk

1 cup whole grain cereal (any brand 150 calories or less per 1 cup serving with 3+ grams fiber) with 1 cup skim milk or light soy milk.

Any HALF serving of fruit

(Tasty options include 1 orange, ½ grapefruit, ½ cup grapes, or 10 strawberries.)

LUNCH

Sicilian Tuna Salad (page 283)

Served on a bed of greens.

Enjoy with 2 plain rice cakes (45 calories or less per cake).

SNACK

1 part-skim stick cheese+small apple (or any HALF fruit serving).

DINNER

LIFE Dinner Salad (page 59)

~ or ~

2 cups *LIFE* Veggie Soup (page 63)

Mini Turkey Meatloaves (page 221)

(2 mini meatloaves)

Cauliflower Mash (page 69)

1 serving (¾ cup)

(Can substitute steamed cauliflower, broccoli, or Brussels sprouts.)

BREAKFAST

English Muffin with Apple Butter

1 whole wheat English muffin, split and lightly toasted. Spread with 1 table-spoon apple butter.

½ cup 1% low-fat or fat-free cottage cheese

(Or substitute any other breakfast protein.)

LUNCH

LIFE Chef's Salad

Unlimited bed of greens topped with sliced turkey breast, lean ham, or roast beef (any combination totaling 4 ounces of meat).

2 hardboiled egg whites and unlimited non-starchy vegetables (tomatoes, carrots, sliced cucumber, etc.).

Dress with 2 tablespoons reduced calorie dressing or 1 teaspoon olive oil with unlimited vinegar.

SNACK

LIFE Muffin (pages 119–123)

DINNER

LIFE Dinner Salad (page 59)

~ or ~

2 cups *LIFE* Veggie Soup (page 63)
Microwave Poached Salmon with Lemon Dill Sauce (page 219)
EZ Garlic Broccoli

Preheat oven to 450°F. Cut one large bunch of broccoli into florets.

Sprinkle with 1 clove minced garlic (1 teaspoon) and season with salt and pepper.

Tightly wrap in aluminum foil and place in oven for 8 to 10 minutes.

BREAKFAST

LIFE Smoothie (pages 132–133)

Choose from Banana Cardamom, Blueberry Mango, Creamsicle, or Strawberry Banana Smoothie.

3 Slices Turkey Bacon

(Or substitute any other breakfast protein.)

LUNCH

Grilled Chicken-Pepper Wrap

Slice 5 ounces boneless skinless chicken breast into strips.

Sauté chicken with unlimited sliced pepper and onion and desired seasonings in pan coated with nonstick cooking spray over medium high heat until cooked through.

Add mixture to center of whole wheat wrap (any wrap 100 calories or less) and fold.

Enjoy with unlimited cucumber slices.

SNACK

4 cups light popcorn (with or without LIFE seasoning options).

DINNER

LIFE Dinner Salad (page 59)

~ or ~

2 cups *LIFE* Veggie Soup (page 63)
Loaded Veggie Frittata (page 226)

BREAKFAST

English Muffin Hawaiian-Style

Combine ¼ cup reduced-fat (part-skim) ricotta cheese (or ½ cup 1% low-fat or fat-free cottage cheese) with a dash of cinnamon and ¼ cup crushed pineapple (packed in its own juice and drained).

Spread evenly on a toasted whole grain English muffin.

LUNCH

Classic Roast Beef Sandwich

Two slices reduced-calorie whole wheat bread with 4 ounces lean roast beef, optional lettuce, tomatoes, onions, and pickles, and mustard, ketchup, or 1 tablespoon reduced-fat or nonfat sour cream mixed with 1 teaspoon horseradish.

Enjoy with baby carrots, celery sticks, and/or cucumber slices.

SNACK

One WHOLE fruit serving.

DINNER

Whole Wheat Pasta with Sausage and Peppers

Prepare one serving Turkey Sausage with Sautéed Peppers and Onions (page 144).

Pour over ½ cup cooked whole wheat spaghetti or penne.

Top with ½ cup heated marinara sauce.

BREAKFAST

Smoked Salmon Omelet (page 214)

LUNCH

Roasted Red Pepper & Mozzarella Melt

Lightly toast 2 slices reduced-calorie whole wheat bread.

Top each slice with roasted red pepper strips (if packed in oil, pat dry) and ¼ cup (1 ounce) shredded or sliced reduced-fat (part-skim) mozzarella cheese.

Place in oven or under broiler until cheese melts.

Serve with plain balsamic vinegar drizzled on top (optional).

Enjoy with unlimited celery sticks, carrots, pepper strips, or other non-starchy vegetable.

SNACK

Naked Turkey/Ham Roll-up

Lay down unlimited large leaves of lettuce (such as Romaine).

Top with 4 ounces turkey breast or lean ham and mustard, roll, and eat with your fingers.

DINNER

Sweet and Sour Chicken (page 228) Over Rice

1 serving (2 cups) over ½ cup cooked brown rice.

BREAKFAST

Breakfast Turkey Melt

Split and lightly toast 1 whole grain English muffin.

Top each half with 1 teaspoon reduced-fat mayo or mustard (optional), 1 ounce turkey breast, and sliced tomato.

Top off each half with 2 tablespoons (½ ounce) shredded reduced-fat cheese.

Place under broiler or in oven until cheese melts.

LUNCH

Breakfast for Lunch: Cereal with Milk

1 cup whole grain cereal (any brand 150 calories or less per 1 cup serving with 3+ grams fiber).

1 cup skim milk or light soy milk.

Any HALF serving of fruit

(Tasty options include 1 orange, ½ grapefruit, ½ cup grapes, or 10 strawberries.)

One hard-boiled egg or 4 egg whites

(Or substitute any other breakfast protein.)

SNACK

Spinach Marinara

Microwave one 10-ounce package of frozen chopped spinach until cooked. Thoroughly drain and mix with 2 heaping tablespoons marinara sauce. Place back in microwave and reheat for 45 seconds. Top with optional 2 table-spoons grated Parmesan or reduced-fat shredded cheese.

DINNER

LIFE Dinner Salad (page 59)

~ or ~

2 cups *LIFE* Veggie Soup (page 63)

Pizza Burger

5 ounce turkey burger, cooked as desired, and topped with ¼ cup heated marinara sauce and one (1 ounce) slice or ¼ cup shredded reduced-fat (part-skim) mozzarella cheese.

*Microwave topped burger for 30 to 60 seconds, or just until cheese melts. Enjoy burger **without** bun.*

BREAKFAST

LIFE Muffin (pages 119–123)

> *Any variety.*

1 cup nonfat plain, Greek, or flavored yogurt

> *Any brand 100 calories or less.*

> *(Or substitute any other breakfast protein.)*

LUNCH

Honey Mustard Chicken Wrap

> *Mix together 1 tablespoon Dijon mustard and 1 teaspoon honey and toss with 4 to 5 ounces cooked chicken breast, shredded or chopped (fresh or canned).*

> *Spoon onto whole wheat wrap (any wrap 100 calories or less) and top with tomato, pepper strips, and lettuce or spinach leaves. Wrap tightly.*

> *Enjoy with baby carrots.*

SNACK

> *Unlimited celery sticks with 4 rounded tablespoons fat-free cream cheese (or 2 rounded tablespoons reduced-fat cream cheese, or 1 level tablespoon peanut butter).*

DINNER

LIFE Dinner Salad (page 59)

~ or ~

2 cups *LIFE* Veggie Soup (page 63)

Ginger Lime Salmon Cakes (pages 224–225)

> *One serving (2 salmon cakes).*

Teriyaki Vegetables

> *Unlimited steamed green beans and red pepper strips topped with*

> *2 tablespoons low-sodium teriyaki sauce and sprinkled with optional 1 teaspoon sesame seeds.*

BREAKFAST

Ricotta Tomato Toast

Lightly toast 2 slices reduced calorie whole wheat bread.

Top each slice with ¼ cup low-fat (part-skim) ricotta cheese and tomato slices. Season with black pepper, garlic powder, and/or dried or fresh herbs.

Place under broiler or in oven until hot.

LUNCH

Chicken, Vegetables, and Potato

5 ounces skinless grilled chicken breast or fish.

Half a medium baked potato (white or sweet), plain or with 2 tablespoons ketchup or salsa.

Unlimited steamed non-starchy vegetables.

SNACK

Vanilla Pumpkin Pudding

6 ounces nonfat vanilla yogurt (any brand 100 calories or less) mixed with ½ cup 100% pure pumpkin puree and cinnamon to taste.

DINNER

LIFE Dinner Salad (page 59)

~ or ~

2 cups *LIFE* Veggie Soup (page 63)
Turkey Tacos (page 227)

2 tacos with toppings.

BREAKFAST

Oatmeal with Fruit and Nuts

Prepare ½ cup dry traditional oatmeal (or ¼ cup steel-cut oats) with water.

Top with any HALF serving of fruit (tasty options include ¾ cup berries or 1 small apple, chopped)

~ and ~

one tablespoon chopped nuts (almonds, walnuts, or pecans) or ground flaxseed.

Optional one teaspoon sugar (white or brown), honey, maple syrup, or artificial sweetener.

LUNCH

Easy Cheesy Salmon Melt (page 283)

SNACK

One WHOLE fruit serving.

DINNER

Gorgonzola-Walnut Stuffed Chicken Breast (page 225)

Roasted Balsamic Asparagus

Preheat oven to 350°F. Assemble asparagus on baking sheet sprayed with nonstick cooking spray.

Drizzle asparagus with 1 to 2 tablespoons balsamic vinegar and season with salt and pepper to taste.

Roast for 20 minutes.

BREAKFAST

Peanut Butter Pita

1 mini whole wheat pita (any brand 70 calories or less per pita).

Spread with 2 level tablespoons peanut, almond, or soy nut butter.

LUNCH

Open-Faced Turkey Picante

Lightly toast 2 slices reduced calorie whole wheat bread.

Top each slice with 2 ounces turkey breast, unlimited roasted red pepper strips, and 1 heaping tablespoon salsa.

Enjoy with unlimited crunchy celery sticks and/or red, yellow, or green pepper strips.

SNACK

Yogurt and Fruit

6 ounces nonfat plain, Greek, or flavored yogurt (any brand 100 calories or less)+HALF fruit serving (e.g., orange, half banana, small apple, ¾ cup berries, or 2 tablespoons raisins).

DINNER

LIFE Dinner Salad (page 59)

~ or ~

2 cups *LIFE* Veggie Soup (page 63)
Lemon Garlic Shrimp (page 224)
Sautéed Mushrooms and Zucchini

Heat medium sauté pan coated with nonstick cooking spray over medium heat.

Sauté 1 small zucchini, sliced into half moons, and ½ cup sliced mushrooms until tender, 6 to 8 minutes.

Season with salt and pepper to taste.

BREAKFAST

English Muffin with Cream Cheese, Tomato, and Lox

Opened-faced, toasted whole grain English muffin (any brand 130 calories or less) with 2 tablespoons reduced-fat or fat-free cream cheese (one tablespoon per slice), unlimited sliced tomato, and 2 ounces sliced lox (one ounce for each slice). Can use 2 slices reduced calorie whole wheat toast (45 calories or less per slice) instead of English muffin. Add sliced onion if desired.

LUNCH

Crab Salad (page 215)

Served over bed of greens
with unlimited sliced cucumber.

SNACK

One WHOLE fruit serving.

DINNER

LIFE Dinner Salad (page 59)

~ or ~

2 cups *LIFE* Veggie Soup (page 63)
Chicken Sloppy Joes (page 225)

1 serving (1¼ cups) Chicken Sloppy Joes served over 2 slices reduced calorie whole wheat bread, lightly toasted

(or, skip the bread and enjoy with ½ medium baked potato, white or sweet).

BREAKFAST

LIFE Bar with Hard Boiled Egg

One Joy Bauer LIFE bar with one hard boiled egg or 4 egg whites.

LUNCH

Chicken Salad with Red Pepper Dippers

Chicken Salad (page 217) with 1 large red (or any other color) pepper, cut into eighths, used to scoop up chicken salad.

Enjoy with any WHOLE fruit serving (tasty options include 1 cup fresh pine-apple chunks, 1 apple, 1 pear, or 1 cup grapes).

SNACK

4 cups low-fat popcorn (with or without LIFE seasoning options).

DINNER

Surf 'n Turf

Shrimp Cocktail

Five large shrimp with 1 heaping tablespoon ketchup + 1 teaspoon horseradish.

Grilled Sirloin Steak

5 ounces lean steak, seasoned as desired with allowed marinades/herbs/ seasonings.

Preheat a large skillet or grill to medium-high heat and cook to preferred temperature.

EZ Garlic Broccoli

Preheat oven to 450°F. Cut one large bunch of broccoli into florets.

Sprinkle with 1 clove minced garlic (1 teaspoon) and season with salt and pepper.

Tightly wrap in aluminum foil and place in oven for 8 to 10 minutes.

BREAKFASTS

Bananas and Cream (Day 1)

Joy Bauer *LIFE* Bar with Yogurt (Day 4)

Fruit, Cheese, and Nuts "To Go" (Day 5)

Yogurt with Fresh Fruit and Wheat Germ (Day 9)

> *Bonus Timesaver: No wheat germ? Skip it completely or add a ¼ cup of any whole grain cereal instead.*

Cereal with Milk and Fruit (Day 10)

English Muffin with Apple Butter and Cottage Cheese (Day 11)

Breakfast Turkey Melt (Day 15)

Peanut Butter Pita (Day 19)

LUNCHES

Ham and Cheese Sandwich (Day 4)

> *Bonus Timesaver: For your side veggies, use baby carrots straight from the bag.*

Steamed Chinese Food (Day 6)

> *Bonus Timesaver: Order takeout. What can be easier?!*

Minestrone Soup and Salad (Day 7)

> *Bonus Timesaver: Use store bought soup (any brand 300 calories or less per two cup serving). For your salad, enjoy a few handfuls of any lettuce blend directly out of the sack. No need to add anything else!*

Classic Roast Beef Sandwich (Day 13)

> *Bonus Timesaver: For your side veggies, use baby carrots straight from the bag.*

Breakfast for Lunch (Day 15)

> *Bonus Timesaver: Swap the hard boiled eggs for a 6-ounce container of nonfat, flavored yogurt or ½ cup nonfat or 1% low-fat cottage cheese.*

(continued)

easiest meals at-a-glance

Open-Faced Turkey Picante (Day 15)

Bonus Timesaver: Leave off the roasted red peppers. Add lettuce and tomato if you have it on hand. For your side veggies, use baby carrots straight from the bag.

DINNERS

Orange Dijon Pork Tenderloin (Day 1)

Bonus Timesaver: Substitute plain steamed or microwave green beans, snow peas, or broccoli for the Green Beans with Tangy Vinaigrette recipe.

Baked Fish with Sautéed Spinach (Day 2)

Bonus Timesaver: Microwave a box frozen chopped spinach in place of sautéed spinach (salt and pepper to taste).

Grilled Sirloin Steak with Tomato Mozzarella Salad (Day 4)

Italian Chicken with Stuffed Portobello Mushroom Caps (Day 8)

Bonus Timesaver: In place of the Stuffed Portobello Mushroom Caps, substitute a LIFE dinner salad with plain balsamic vinegar or 2 tablespoons reduced calorie dressing (40 calories or less per 2 tablespoons).

Steak Balsamica with Oven Roasted Parmesan Cauliflower (Day 9)

Bonus Timesaver: Substitute plain steamed or microwave cauliflower or broccoli for the Oven Roasted Parmesan cauliflower.

Pizza Burger (Day 15)

Bonus Timesaver: Purchase frozen turkey burgers or fresh ground turkey already formed into patties.

easiest meals at-a-glance

Joy's LIFE Diet Step Three Restaurant Options

Some Step Three menu options (as well as menus from Steps One and Two) can easily be ordered in a restaurant, as long as you are willing to make a few special requests about how the foods are prepared. But there are also some generic meals you can order anytime and nearly anywhere. (Always remember: If it is not listed here or in the Unlimited Foods list, don't eat it! For example, don't eat extra bread, rice, fruit, full-fat salad dressings, sauces, etc., unless you're counting toward your *LIFE* Extras). You'll also notice Step Three allows the option of incorporating occasional fast food.

Breakfast

Option #1: Egg white omelet stuffed with any of your favorite vegetables (no cheese—most restaurants don't carry reduced-fat cheese), *plus* ½ grapefruit, or ¼ cantaloupe, or side portion of fresh berries or fruit salad, or one slice dry whole wheat toast.

Option #2: One hard boiled egg (or a side of scrambled egg whites with chopped tomatoes)+one cup plain oatmeal. Top oatmeal with a few tablespoons of berries *or* 1 teaspoon/packet sugar. Artificial sweetener is optional.

Option #3: Scrambled egg whites with chopped tomatoes and herbs + one slice dry whole wheat toast.

For all options, add beverage: Coffee (black, or with skim or 1% milk only) or tea (iced or hot, unsweetened, with lemon *or* skim or 1% milk only). Artificial sweetener optional.

Lunch

Option #1: Large salad piled with assorted raw vegetables and topped with skinless grilled chicken *or* turkey *or* fish/seafood (no cheese). Use plain balsamic vinegar or fresh lemon as dressing, or 2 tablespoons low-calorie dressing (if available).

Option #2: Turkey burger, no bun, with lettuce, tomato, onion, pickles, and optional ketchup. Enjoy your burger with plain raw or steamed vegetables. Or, with a vegetable salad dressed with plain vinegar or fresh lemon or low-fat dressing.

Option #3: Turkey, ham, skinless chicken, or roast beef sandwich on ONE slice whole wheat bread (remove top slice and enjoy open-faced)—enjoy with any of the following toppings; lettuce, tomato, roasted peppers, pickles, onion, and mustard—plus, the option for plain nonstarchy vegetables on the side.

Option #4: One bowl of any non-creamy vegetable-based soup (lentil, black bean, vegetable, or minestrone) along with a plain mixed vegetable salad (omit cheese, croutons, dried fruit, nuts, whole egg and other high-calorie salad ingredients). Dress the salad with plain vinegar, fresh lemon, or 2 tablespoons low-calorie dressing.

For all options, add beverage: Water, seltzer, coffee (black, or with skim or 1% milk only), and/or tea (iced or hot, unsweetened, with lemon *or* skim or 1% milk only). Artificial sweetener optional.

Dinner

OPTION #1: STANDARD RESTAURANT

House salad with plain vinegar or fresh lemon.

Skinless chicken breast *or* fish *or* seafood *or* pork tenderloin *or* turkey *or* lean steak (all options must be grilled, baked, roasted, poached, steamed, or boiled *only*).

Double order of steamed, plain vegetables.

OPTION #2: STEAK HOUSE

Shrimp cocktail with cocktail sauce and lemon

Sliced tomatoes and onion with plain balsamic vinegar (*not* balsamic "vinaigrette")

Grilled or broiled lean steak (sirloin or filet mignon are good options)

Steamed broccoli, spinach or green beans (add lemon, salt and pepper to taste)

OPTION #3: CHINESE FOOD

Cup of soup (choose either egg drop or hot and sour soup or wonton broth without wontons or noodles)

Order "steamed" chicken, shrimp or tofu with vegetables. Request garlic sauce on the side and drizzle ONLY one tablespoon on your steamed entrée (you may add additional low-sodium soy sauce). Avoid all extras including rice, dumplings, noodles, wontons, etc.

OPTION #4: *JAPANESE FOOD (3 CHOICES)*

Teriyaki Dinner:

Miso soup+Chicken or Salmon Teriyaki with Vegetables. Omit the rice and ask the waiter to double up on vegetables.

Sushi Dinner:

Miso soup+house salad (hold the dressing and use soy sauce instead)+one six piece California roll (optional ginger, wasabi, soy sauce)

Sashimi Dinner:

Miso soup+order of edamame (soybeans in the pod)+unlimited sashimi (fish without the rice) (optional ginger, wasabi, and soy sauce). Optional side of steamed vegetables.

For all options, add beverage: Water, seltzer, tea (iced or hot, unsweetened, with lemon *or* skim or 1% milk only). Great after-dinner choices include all herbal teas (especially mint or chamomile) and green tea. Artificial sweetener optional.

LIFE Fast Food Options

Although fast food is typically not the best choice (and should only be eaten occasionally), we're sometimes faced with no option or simply have an irresistible craving. If that's the case, enjoy the following LIFE selections for breakfast, lunch, or dinner. To date, these items are available and meet the calorie requirements for your Step Three food plan. To access additional fast food and restaurant options, and check the status of menu revisions for each chain, go to www.JoyBauer.com.

BURGER KING

Lunch Options

Tendergrill Chicken Garden Salad (with 1 packet KEN'S Fat-free Ranch dressing *or* ½ packet KEN'S Light Italian dressing)

BK Veggie Burger (without cheese + request no mayo)

Whopper Jr. Sandwich (without cheese + request no mayo)

*Dinner Options**

Tendergrill Chicken Sandwich (request no mayo)

Tendergrill Chicken Garden Salad (with 1 packet KEN'S Fat-free Ranch dressing *or* ½ packet KEN'S Light Italian dressing)

BK Veggie Burger (request no mayo) + **side garden salad** (with 1 packet KEN'S Fat-free Ranch dressing *or* ½ packet KEN'S Light Italian dressing)

Whopper Jr. Sandwich (request no mayo) + **side garden salad** (with 1 packet KEN'S Fat-free Ranch dressing *or* ½ packet KEN'S Light Italian dressing)

*You may also enjoy any of the lunch options for dinner.

MCDONALD'S

Breakfast Options

Scrambled Eggs (2), plain

One Scrambled Egg on English Muffin

Fruit 'n' Yogurt Parfait with granola

Fruit & Walnut Salad, snack size

Lunch Options

Premium Asian Salad with grilled chicken (with 1 packet Newman's Own Low-fat Balsamic Vinaigrette or Low-fat Italian dressing)

Premium Southwest Salad with grilled chicken (with 1 packet Newman's Own Low-fat Balsamic Vinaigrette or Low-fat Italian dressing)

Premium Bacon Ranch Salad with grilled chicken (with 1 packet Newman's Own Low-fat Balsamic Vinaigrette or Low-fat Italian dressing)

Premium Caesar Salad with grilled chicken and bag of croutons (with 1 packet Newman's Own Low-fat Balsamic Vinaigrette or Low-fat Italian dressing)

1 Snack Wrap with grilled chicken: Ranch, Honey Mustard, or Chipotle BBQ flavor + **garden salad** (with 1 packet Newman's Own Low-fat Balsamic Vinaigrette or Low-fat Italian dressing)

Plain Hamburger on bun (with lettuce, tomato, onion, ketchup and pickles) + **garden salad** (with 1 packet Newman's Own Low-fat Balsamic Vinaigrette or Low-fat Italian dressing)

6-piece Chicken McNuggets with 2 ketchup packets+garden side salad (with 1 packet Newman's Own Low-fat Balsamic Vinaigrette or Low-fat Italian dressing)

Premium Grilled Chicken Classic Sandwich (with lettuce, tomato, pickles, onion, ketchup, and mustard; request no mayo)

* You may also enjoy any of the listed lunch salads and appropriate dressings for dinner.

LIFE Extras (150 calories or less)

1 kiddie size vanilla reduced-fat ice cream cone

1 oatmeal raisin or sugar cookie

2 bags apple dippers with 1 tub low-fat caramel dip

WENDY'S

Lunch Options

Plain baked potato+side salad (with 1 packet fat-free French, light Honey Dijon, light Classic Ranch, or Balsamic Vinaigrette dressing)

Large chili+side salad (with 1 packet fat-free French, light Honey Dijon, light Classic Ranch, or Balsamic Vinaigrette dressing)

Small chili+1 packet of saltine crackers+side salad (with 1 packet fat-free French, light Honey Dijon, light Classic Ranch, or Balsamic Vinaigrette dressing)

Ultimate Chicken Grill Sandwich (with lettuce, tomato, ketchup, pickles, onions, and mustard; request no mayo)

5-piece Crispy Chicken Nuggets with ketchup+side salad (with 1 packet fat-free French, light Honey Dijon, light Classic Ranch, or Balsamic Vinaigrette dressing)

Dinner Options*

1 Single (¼ lb) Hamburger (with lettuce, tomato, ketchup, pickles, onions, and mustard; request no mayo)

1 Jr. Hamburger+small chili

1 Jr. Hamburger+side salad (with 1 packet fat-free French, light Honey Dijon, light Classic Ranch, or Balsamic Vinaigrette dressing)

Ultimate Chicken Grill Sandwich (request no mayo)+**side salad** (with 1 packet fat-free French, light Honey Dijon, light Classic Ranch, or Balsamic Vinaigrette dressing)

Ultimate Chicken Grill Sandwich (request no mayo)+**Mandarin Orange Cup**

Mandarin Chicken Salad (with 1 packet fat-free French, light Honey Dijon, light Classic Ranch, or Balsamic Vinaigrette dressing)

Chicken Caesar Salad (with 1 packet fat-free French, light Honey Dijon, light Classic Ranch, or Balsamic Vinaigrette dressing)

Double Stack Sandwich (request no mayo)

Jr. Cheeseburger Deluxe (request no mayo)

Plain baked potato+broccoli+reduced-fat sour cream (request no butter on potato)

* You may also enjoy any of the lunch options for dinner.

LIFE Extras (150 calories or less)

Jr. size vanilla or chocolate Frosty

PANERA BREAD

Breakfast Options

Half whole grain bagel+1 oz serving reduced-fat plain cream cheese

Half egg and cheese grilled breakfast sandwich

Lunch Options

Half Mediterranean Veggie Sandwich on tomato basil bread

Half Smoked Turkey Breast Sandwich on whole grain or sourdough bread+small fruit cup

Half Smoked Turkey Breast Sandwich on whole grain or sourdough bread+1 cup (8 oz) serving low-fat chicken noodle soup or vegetarian garden vegetable soup

1 cup (8 oz) serving low-fat chicken noodle, vegetarian garden vegetable soup, or black bean soup+any slice of bread or small roll (preferably whole grain)

Classic Café Salad with grilled chicken with light, fat-free, or fat-free reduced sugar dressing (no bread)

Half Mediterranean Veggie on tomato basil bread + 1 cup (8 oz) serving low-fat chicken noodle soup or vegetarian garden vegetable soup, or small fruit cup

Full Asian Sesame Chicken Salad (with light, fat-free, or fat-free reduced sugar dressing)

Full Fandango Salad (with light, fat-free, or fat-free reduced sugar dressing)

Half Grilled Chicken Caesar Salad (with light, fat-free, or fat-free reduced sugar dressing)

* You may also enjoy any of the lunch options for dinner.

LIFE Extras (150 calories or less)

2 oz serving of any Artisan Bread (except focaccia and focaccia with asiago cheese)

2 oz serving of french loaf, sourdough loaf, sourdough XL loaf, tomato basil loaf, or white whole grain loaf

1 petite cookie (any flavor)

1 cup (8 oz) serving low-fat chicken noodle, low-fat vegetarian garden vegetable, or low-fat vegetarian black bean soup

SUBWAY

Breakfast Option

2 packages of apple slices + 1 Dannon All Natural Strawberry yogurt

Lunch Options

The following toppings may be enjoyed on any listed lunch or dinner sandwich/wrap option: lettuce, onion, peppers (sweet or hot), tomatoes, olives, pickles, ketchup, mustard, and vinegar.

Veggie Delight wrap

6" Veggie Delight on wheat bun

6" Oven Roasted Chicken Breast on wheat bun

6" Roast Beef on wheat bun

6" Turkey Breast on wheat bun

6" Turkey Breast and Ham on wheat bun

Dinner Options*

Roast Beef wrap

Ham wrap

Turkey wrap

6" Sweet Onion Teriyaki on wheat bun

* You may also enjoy any of the listed lunch options for dinner with 1 package of apple slices *or* 1 Dannon All Natural Strawberry yogurt (optional).

TACO BELL

Lunch Options

2 Fresco Crunchy Tacos

2 Fresco Beef *or* **Ranchero Chicken** *or* **Grilled Steak Soft Tacos**

1 Fresco Zesty Chicken Border Bowl (without dressing)

1 Fresco (Chicken or Steak) Burrito Supreme

1 Fresco Fiesta Burrito—chicken

1 Fresco Bean Burrito

1 Gordita—any variety

Dinner Options*

1 Double Decker Taco Supreme

1 Chalupa—any variety

1 Burrito Supreme—chicken or steak

1 Spicy Chicken Burrito

* You may also enjoy any of the lunch options for dinner.

STARBUCKS

Breakfast Options

Fruit cup+Skinny Latte (Tall, Grande or Venti)

Perfect Oatmeal *with only one of the following toppings*: **Nut Medley** *or* **brown sugar** *or* **dried fruit+black coffee** (with optional skim milk)

Chewy Fruit & Nut Bar+black coffee (with optional skim milk)

Grande (16 oz) Vivanno Orange Mango Banana Blend

Spinach, Roasted Tomato, Feta, & Egg Wrap+black coffee (with optional skim milk)

JAMBA JUICE

Breakfast Options

One 16 oz serving of any of the following flavors:

Strawberry Whirl

Mega Mango

Peach Perfection

Jamba Light Berry Fulfilling

Jamba Light Mango Mantra

Jamba Light Strawberry Nirvana

BOSTON MARKET

Dinner Options

Roasted Turkey Breast (no skin)+side order garlic dill new potatoes+fresh steamed veggies

¼ White Rotisserie Chicken (no skin)+side order garlic dill new potatoes+fresh steamed veggies

Half Boston Chicken Carver Sandwich+fresh steamed veggies

3-piece Dark Skinless Rotisserie Chicken (thigh+2 drumsticks)+fresh steamed veggies

DOMINO'S PIZZA

Lunch or Dinner Options

1 slice of 14-inch (large) crunchy thin crust pizza (plain cheese *or* topped with green peppers, onions and mushrooms)+½ container garden fresh salad (with 1 packet light Italian dressing)

2 slices of 12-inch (medium) crunchy thin crust pizza (plain cheese *or* topped with green peppers, onions and mushrooms)+½ container garden fresh salad (with 1 packet light Italian dressing)

LIFE Extras (150 calories or less)

1 slice of 12-inch (medium) crunchy thin crust pizza (plain cheese *or* topped with green peppers, onions and mushrooms)

1 slice 12-inch (medium) crunchy thin crust pizza topped with ham and pineapple

PANDA EXPRESS Gourmet Chinese Food

Lunch or Dinner Options

(12 oz) **Hot and Sour Soup**+(5.5 oz) **Tangy Shrimp**+(5.5 oz) **Mixed Veggies**

(12 oz) **Hot and Sour Soup**+(5.5 oz) **Broccoli Beef**+(5.5 oz) **Mixed Veggies**

KFC

Dinner Option

2 pieces **Oven-Roasted Chicken Breast** (without skin and breading)+**side of green beans**+**one 3" corn on the cob**

HARDEE'S

Breakfast Option

1 **folded egg**+**side order of grits**+**1 slice country ham**

Lunch Options

Hamburger on bun (with lettuce, tomato, onion, pickles, ketchup, and mustard; request no mayo)

BBQ Chicken Sandwich (request no mayo)

*Dinner Options**

Cheeseburger on bun (with lettuce, tomato, onion, pickles, ketchup, and mustard; request no mayo)

Low Carb Charbroiled Chicken Club Sandwich (request no mayo)

* You may also enjoy any of the lunch options for dinner.

CHICK-FIL-A

Lunch Options

Chargrilled Chicken Sandwich on bun (with lettuce, tomato, onion, pickles, ketchup, and mustard; request no mayo)

Chargrilled Chicken Garden Salad (with 1 packet light Italian dressing)+**1 fruit cup**

Chargrilled Chicken & Fruit Salad (with 1 packet light Italian dressing)

Hearty Breast of Chicken Soup+**1 fruit cup**

*Dinner Options**

Chargrilled Chicken Sandwich on bun (with lettuce, tomato, onion, pickles, ketchup, and mustard; request no mayo)**+1 fruit cup**

Southwest Chargrilled Salad (with 1 packet light Italian dressing)**+1 fruit cup**

Spicy Chicken Cool Wrap

Chicken Salad Cup+1 side Salad (no dressing)

* You may also enjoy any lunch option for dinner.

CHIPOTLE

For salsa options listed, choose from: Fresh Tomato, Tomatillo-Green Chili, or Tomatillo-Red Chili. You may also add lettuce to any entrée.

Lunch Options

Salad with Steak or Barbacoa+salsa+one of the following choices: beans or guacamole

Salad with choice of meat+salsa+one of the following choices: fajita veggies, cheese, or sour cream

Salad with beans+salsa+one of the following choices: guacamole, rice, sour cream, cheese, or fajita veggies

Salad with fajita veggies+salsa+one of the following choices: guacamole, rice, beans, sour cream, or cheese

Salad with rice+salsa+one of the following choices: guacamole, beans, sour cream, cheese, or fajita veggies

Crispy taco shells (3 per order)**+salsa+one of the following choices: fajita veggies or beans**

*Dinner Options**

Salad with choice of meat+salsa+one of the following choices: beans, guacamole, or rice

Salad with fajita veggies+salsa+sour cream *or* **cheese+one of the following choices: beans, guacamole, or rice**

Crispy taco shells (3 per order)**+salsa+fajita veggies+cheese**

Crispy taco shells (3 per order)**+salsa+choice of meat**

Burrito flour tortilla *or* **taco flour tortillas** (3 per order)**+salsa+fajita veggies**

* You may also enjoy any lunch option for dinner.

FIESTA SCRAMBLED EGGS WITH GREEN CHILES

1 whole egg

3 egg whites

1 tablespoon diced green chiles, canned

2 tablespoons reduced-fat cheddar cheese

1 tablespoon low-fat or nonfat sour cream

2 tablespoons salsa (optional)

Heat pan coated with nonstick cooking spray over medium heat. Whip eggs with green chiles and a splash of water (for fluffier eggs). Pour eggs into a pan and scramble. Top with cheese and cook an for additional 30 seconds, or until cheese is melted. Transfer to a plate. Top with sour cream and salsa.

Makes one serving

VANILLA FRENCH TOAST

2 large egg whites

1 tablespoon skim milk

2 teaspoons sugar or equivalent amount of artificial sweetener (optional)

½ teaspoon vanilla extract

¼ teaspoon cinnamon

Pinch of nutmeg

2 slices reduced calorie whole wheat bread

Whip together egg whites with milk, sugar, vanilla, cinnamon, and nutmeg. Soak bread in egg mixture. Heat a nonstick pan coated with cooking spray over medium heat. Fry bread slices until crispy on both sides.

Makes one serving

SMOKED SALMON OMELET

1 whole egg

3 egg whites

2 ounces smoked salmon, cut into strips

Preferred seasonings

2 tablespoons low-fat or nonfat sour cream

1 teaspoon minced chives or small pinch dried dill weed

Heat a pan sprayed with nonstick cooking spray over medium heat. Whip the eggs and pour into the pan. Sprinkle in the salmon. Add the seasonings and continue to cook. When the bottom side is cooked, gently flip and cook the other side. Fold one side over the other. Top with a dollop of sour cream blended with chives or dill weed.

Makes one serving

SPINACH AND FETA EGG SCRAMBLE

1 whole egg

3 egg whites

1 to 2 cups fresh spinach leaves

Preferred seasonings

1 ounce feta cheese (approximately 3 tablespoons crumbled) or 1 ounce reduced-fat cheese

Heat a pan coated with nonstick cooking spray over medium heat. Add the spinach and sauté until cooked down, 3 to 5 minutes. Whip the eggs with desired seasonings and a splash of water (for fluffier eggs). Pour into the pan and scramble with the spinach. Transfer to a plate and top with the feta cheese.

Makes one serving

EGG WHITE SALAD

1 tablespoon reduced-fat mayo

1 tablespoon 1% low-fat or fat-free cottage cheese

1 teaspoon Dijon mustard

4 large egg whites, hardboiled

1 rib of celery, chopped

1 scallion, chopped, or fresh thyme, chives, or onion

¼ apple, peeled and chopped

Black pepper

In a small bowl, combine the mayo, cottage cheese, and mustard. Chop the egg whites and add to the mayo mixture, along with the celery, scallions, and apple. Stir to combine. Season with black pepper to taste.

Makes one serving

CRAB SALAD

6 to 8 ounces crab or imitation crab meat (fresh or frozen)

2 teaspoons lemon juice

Zest of ½ lemon (optional)

2 tablespoons reduced-fat mayo

Good pinch Old Bay seasoning

2 tablespoons red onion, finely chopped

Black pepper

Combine all the ingredients.

Makes one serving

SICILIAN TUNA SALAD

1 (6-ounce) can chunk light tuna in water, drained

6 green olives, chopped

1 to 2 teaspoons capers with juices (optional)

1 rib celery, diced

1 to 2 tablespoons diced red onion

1 teaspoon olive oil

1 tablespoon lemon juice

Black pepper

Mash tuna with olives, capers, celery, and onion. Add olive oil, lemon juice, and pepper and toss to coat.

Makes one serving

EASY CHEESY SALMON MELT

4 ounces boneless, skinless wild salmon, drained and mashed

1 tablespoon reduced-fat mayo

1 teaspoon lemon juice

Black pepper to taste

1 ounce shredded reduced-fat cheese (recommended: cheddar)

2 slices reduced calorie whole wheat bread, lightly toasted

Mash together the salmon, mayo, lemon juice, and pepper. Divide the mixture and spread over the bread. Sprinkle the cheese over two slices. Place under preheated broiler for 3 to 4 minutes or until the cheese melts and the top is golden brown.

Makes one serving

CHICKEN SALAD

4 to 5 ounces cooked chicken breast, shredded or chopped (fresh or canned)

1 tablespoon reduced-fat mayo

1 tablespoon low-fat or nonfat sour cream

1 rib celery, finely chopped

2 tablespoons finely chopped onion (optional)

Black pepper to taste

Pinch of garlic powder and/or onion powder (optional)

Thoroughly mix all the ingredients together.

Makes one serving

GREEK SALAD WITH FETA

Unlimited bed of salad greens

2 ounces feta cheese (about 6 tablespoons crumbled)

10 pitted olives

1 medium tomato, cut into wedges

½ small red onion, sliced

1 teaspoon olive oil

Unlimited red wine vinegar

Pinch of oregano

Top salad greens with feta cheese, olives, and vegetables. Drizzle with olive oil and vinegar; sprinkle with oregano.

Makes one serving

LIFE SCALLION PANCAKE WITH SOUR CREAM

½ cup quick-cooking (plain) oatmeal, dry (do not use steel-cut oats)

4 egg whites, whipped

¼ to ½ cup chopped scallions

1 ounce reduced-fat shredded cheddar cheese

Pinch of salt and pepper

2 heaping tablespoons low-fat or nonfat sour cream

Thoroughly whip together the oatmeal, egg whites, scallions, cheese, salt, and pepper to taste. Preheat a pan coated with nonstick cooking spray over medium heat. Pour in the batter and spread evenly throughout pan. Cook for 2 to 3 minutes (for a moister pancake, cover the pan with a lid while cooking). When golden brown, flip and cook the other side. (This prepares one large pancake; you may choose to make 2 to 3 small pancakes instead.) Top pancake(s) with the sour cream.

Makes one serving

Recipes—Dinners and Sides

CREAMY COLESLAW FOR ONE

3 tablespoons nonfat plain yogurt or nonfat sour cream

2 teaspoons cider vinegar

1 teaspoon sugar

⅛ teaspoon celery seed

Salt and pepper

2 cups bagged coleslaw mix

½ small bell pepper (any color), sliced into thin strips

Mix together the yogurt, vinegar, sugar, celery seed, salt, and pepper. Toss with the coleslaw mix and bell pepper. Enjoy immediately, or refrigerate for at least 2 hours before serving for a soggier slaw.

Makes one serving

MICROWAVE POACHED SALMON WITH LEMON DILL SAUCE

Poached Salmon:

> *½ cup water*
>
> *¼ cup dry white wine*
>
> *Juice of ½ lemon*
>
> *1 bay leaf*
>
> *½ teaspoon ground black pepper*
>
> *1 clove garlic, minced (or ¼ teaspoon garlic powder)*
>
> *4 tablespoons chopped onion*
>
> *6 ounce salmon fillet*

Lemon Dill Sauce:

> *2 tablespoons low-fat or nonfat sour cream*
>
> *⅛ teaspoon dried dill weed*
>
> *Squeeze of lemon juice (from reserved lemon half)*
>
> *Ground black pepper to taste*

Combine water, wine, lemon juice, bay leaf, pepper, onion, and garlic in a microwave-safe dish. Microwave on high until the poaching liquid comes to a full boil. Add the salmon to the poaching liquid, cover with plastic wrap, prick plastic wrap, and microwave for 3 to 5 minutes or until the fish is opaque. Remove from the poaching liquid and let stand 2 to 3 minutes before serving.

Combine all the sauce ingredients in a small bowl and dollop onto the cooked salmon.

Makes one serving

CRISPY OVEN FRIED COD

> *2 tablespoons bread crumbs (preferably whole wheat)*
>
> *1½ teaspoons lemon juice*
>
> *1 teaspoon Dijon mustard*
>
> *1 tablespoon chopped fresh herbs, such as chives, parsley, tarragon, or dill (optional)*

Salt and pepper

6 ounce cod fillet (or other white flaky fish such as tilapia, haddock, or flounder)

Preheat the oven to 400°F. In a small bowl, toss together the bread crumbs, lemon juice, mustard, herbs, salt, and pepper. Lightly season the fish with salt and pepper and place on a baking sheet prepared with nonstick cooking spray. Press the bread crumb topping mixture over the top of the fish. Mist the bread crumb topping with a nonstick cooking spray. Bake for 12 to 16 minutes, or until the topping is crispy and the fish is opaque and cooked through.

Makes one serving

CURRY SWEET POTATO FRIES

1 medium sweet potato

½ teaspoon curry powder

Salt and pepper to taste

Preheat the oven to 400°F. Cut the sweet potato in half, then cut each half into wedges or strips (approximately ¼ inch thick). Spray a baking sheet with nonstick cooking spray. Spread out fries on the baking sheet and spray them liberally with nonstick cooking spray. Sprinkle with curry powder, salt, and pepper. Toss the fries with hands to coat evenly with the seasonings, then arrange the fries in a single layer. Bake for 20 minutes, flipping the fries halfway through. To finish, set the oven to broil and broil for 5 or more minutes (depending on how brown and crispy you like your fries).

Makes 2 servings

MINI TURKEY MEATLOAVES

1 yellow onion, diced

1 red pepper, diced

2 stalks celery, diced

2 carrots, peeled and grated

1 pound lean ground turkey or chicken

2 egg whites

1 teaspoon ground thyme

½ teaspoon rubbed (ground) sage

1 tablespoon Worcestershire sauce

½ teaspoon salt

½ teaspoon pepper

¼ cup ketchup

8 bay leaves (optional)

Preheat the oven to 425°F. Prepare a standard 12-cup muffin tray with nonstick cooking spray and set aside.

Coat a large nonstick sauté pan with cooking spray and sauté the onion for about 5 minutes over medium heat. Add the peppers, celery, and carrots, and sauté for an additional 8 to 10 minutes. Remove the veggies from heat and allow to cool to room temperature.

In a large bowl, add the ground meat, egg whites, cooled vegetables, thyme, sage, Worcestershire sauce, salt, and pepper. Using your hands, mush ingredients together until they are fully incorporated.

Allot the seasoned meat mixture into 8 muffin cups, smoothing the top of each mini-meatloaf to make it level. Coat each mini meatloaf with ketchup and apply a bay leaf. Bake for 20 to 25 minutes.

Cooked mini meatloaves may be frozen for up to 2 months.

Makes 4 servings, 2 mini meatloaves per serving

UNCLE ONION'S TURKEY BEAN CHILI

1¼ pounds ground turkey (at least 90% lean)

12 ounces crushed tomato (without paste)

12 ounces water

1 large onion, coarsely chopped

2 tablespoons chili powder

1 teaspoon garlic powder

1 teaspoon paprika

Salt

1 teaspoon black pepper

1 teaspoon cumin

1 teaspoon dried oregano

¼ teaspoon ground red pepper (or more for hotter chili)

2 teaspoons all purpose flour

1 can (15 ounces) red kidney beans, rinsed and well drained

In a large skillet over medium-high heat, brown the turkey, stirring to break up the meat. Drain the fat. Add the tomatoes, water, onion, chili powder, garlic powder, paprika, salt to taste, black pepper, cumin, oregano, and red pepper. Mix thoroughly. Cover and simmer, stirring occasionally, for 20 to 22 minutes.

Add in the flour and beans, stirring for 1 minute. Cook uncovered for 10 to 12 minutes, stirring occasionally.

Makes 4 servings, 1½ cups each

FISH FILLET EN PAPILLOTE WITH GARDEN VEGETABLES

1 cup fresh spinach leaves

1 large shallot, thinly sliced

¼ cup mushrooms, thinly sliced

2 thin slices of a large tomato

1 teaspoon dried basil (or ¼ cup fresh basil leaves)

1 thin 5- to 6-ounce fish fillet (good options include flounder, snapper, and sole)

Salt and pepper to taste

2 tablespoons sherry (can substitute dry white wine)

Preheat the oven to 400°F. Lay a 15 by 15-inch sheet of parchment or foil flat on the countertop. Layer the spinach leaves in the center, sprinkle with half of the shallots and mushrooms, and top with 1 tomato slice. Sprinkle the veggies with ½ teaspoon dried basil (or half of the fresh basil leaves). Lay the fish fillet on top and season with salt and pepper. Place the remaining mushrooms and shallots on top of the fillet, lay the remaining tomato slice on top, and season with salt, pepper, and the remaining basil. Pour the sherry over all.

Gather two sides of the parchment or foil, double the sides up and fold together, creasing several times, to make a seal down the center of the packet. Fold each open end under the packet, creasing several times to secure.

Place on the baking sheet and bake for 12 to 15 minutes, or until the fish flakes easily when tested with a fork. To serve, tear or cut open the packet carefully, taking care not to get burned by the steam.

Makes one serving

LEMON GARLIC SHRIMP

8 ounces raw shrimp

1 clove garlic, minced (1 teaspoon) or ¼ teaspoon garlic powder

1 teaspoon dried basil (or 2 tablespoons chopped fresh basil)

1 lemon (cut one half of the lemon into thin slices, reserve the other half for juicing)

1 tablespoon Dijon mustard

Salt and pepper to taste

Preheat the oven to 350°F. In a large bowl, toss together the shrimp, garlic, basil, juice of half a lemon, mustard, and salt and pepper to taste, making sure that the shrimp are evenly coated. Place a 12 by 16-inch aluminum foil sheet flat on the countertop. Lay lemon slices in the center, top with the shrimp mixture. Wrap securely, making sure to seal the top and ends of the packet. Place on the baking sheet and bake for 20 minutes.

Makes one serving

GINGER LIME SALMON CAKES

¼ cup oats, old-fashioned or quick-cooking (not steel cut)

¼ cup skim milk

2 tablespoons finely chopped fresh cilantro

2 teaspoons minced or grated fresh ginger

2 scallions, finely chopped

1 egg white

1 lime, juiced and zested (zest optional)

Black pepper to taste

1 (14¾ ounce) can boneless, skinless wild salmon, drained

Preheat oven to 350°F. In a medium bowl, mix together the oats and milk and soak for about 30 minutes. Add the cilantro, ginger, scallions, egg white, lime juice and zest, and black pepper to the mik/oat mixture and stir to combine. Add the salmon and stir gently, but thoroughly, to mix. The mixture will be on the wet side, but will bind up when cooked. Place a large sauté pan coated with nonstick cooking spray over medium heat. Gently shape the salmon mixture into 6 cakes and place in a preheated sauté pan. (Cook in two batches of 3 cakes if you don't have a large enough pan to accommodate 6 cakes.) Cook, flipping once, until cakes are golden brown on both sides and firm to the touch.

Makes 3 servings, 2 cakes each

CHICKEN SLOPPY JOES

1 pound ground chicken (at least 90% lean)

2 cloves garlic, minced (2 teaspoons)

1 small onion, diced

1 green pepper, chopped

1 medium zucchini, chopped

1 large tomato, or 2 small tomatoes, chopped

½ cup chili sauce

½ cup tomato juice (preferably low-sodium)

¼ cup cider vinegar

1 tablespoon chili powder

Salt and pepper to taste

Cover a large fry pan with cooking spray and place over medium heat. Add the ground chicken and sauté until thoroughly cooked, 5 to 10 minutes. Add all the remaining ingredients, mixing thoroughly. Reduce heat to low and simmer, uncovered, for 20 minutes.

Makes 4 servings, 1¼ cups each

GORGONZOLA-WALNUT STUFFED CHICKEN BREAST

2 tablespoons gorgonzola cheese

½ small shallot, minced (about 1 tablespoon)

1 level tablespoon chopped walnuts

¼ cup cooked spinach (from fresh or frozen), chopped, cooled to room temperature

1 (6 ounce) boneless, skinless chicken breast

Salt and pepper

Preheat the oven to 350°F. Place the gorgonzola, shallot, walnuts, and spinach in a bowl. Season lightly with salt and pepper and mash together. Clean and trim the chicken breast. Holding the breast flat, slice sideways, being careful not to cut through to the other side. Fill the chicken breast with stuffing, adding small amounts at a time and filling liberally. Coat a fry pan with cooking spray and heat to medium high. Season the chicken with salt and pepper, sear in the pan until brown on one side, then turn and sear quickly on the other side. Place the chicken on a baking sheet sprayed with nonstick cooking spray. Bake for 20 to 25 minutes to finish cooking the chicken.

Makes one serving

LOADED VEGGIE FRITTATA

2 tablespoons chopped onion (¼ of a small to medium onion)

1 cup broccoli, chopped (fresh or thawed from frozen)

½ medium red bell pepper, chopped

3 large egg whites

1 whole large egg

2 plum tomatoes, chopped

1 scallion, chopped

Salt and pepper

1 ounce shredded reduced-fat sharp cheddar cheese

Preheat the oven to 400°F. Heat an 8 to 10-inch oven-proof skillet* sprayed with nonstick cooking spray over medium heat. Add the onion, broccoli, and pepper and sauté until tender, 5 to 7 minutes. Whisk together the eggs in a medium bowl, then stir in the chopped tomatoes and scallions and season to taste with salt and pepper. Pour the egg/tomato/scallion mixture over the sautéed veggies. Bake for 20 minutes, or until the frittata is puffed and golden and firm in the center. Add the shredded cheese and return to the oven for 3 to 5 minutes, until the cheese is just melted.

* If you do not own an oven-proof skillet, transfer the cooked veggies to a 9-inch pie plate or similarly sized baking dish sprayed with nonstick cooking spray. Pour the egg/tomato/scallion mixture over the top and bake as directed above.

Makes one serving

TURKEY TACOS

1 pound ground turkey (at least 90% lean)

1 packet (1¼ to 1½ ounces) taco seasoning, mild or hot, plus water as indicated
  on the package

2 cups chopped or shredded lettuce

1 large tomato, finely chopped

1 cup shredded reduced-fat cheddar cheese

8 hard or soft taco shells

Salsa and/or hot sauce (optional)

In a large skillet, cook the turkey over medium-high heat until browned. Drain the fat. Stir in the taco seasoning and water. Bring to a boil. Reduce the heat to medium-low and simmer, stirring occasionally, 5 to 6 minutes. Evenly divide the turkey mixture, lettuce, tomato, and cheese among the taco shells. Top with salsa and/or hot sauce.

Makes 8 tacos (2 per serving)

STUFFED PORTOBELLO MUSHROOM CAPS

2 large Portobello mushroom caps, stems removed

½ cup chopped roasted red peppers (if packed in oil, pat dry)

¼ cup shredded reduced-fat (part-skim) mozzarella cheese

⅛ teaspoon dried oregano

Preheat oven to 425°F. Spray mushroom caps with nonstick cooking spray and season with salt and pepper. Place mushrooms, gill sides up, on a baking sheet sprayed with nonstick cooking spray. Roast in the oven for 12 to 15 minutes, until soft and browned. Fill each cap with half of the roasted red peppers. Top each cap with half of the shredded cheese and sprinkle with oregano. Return to the oven for 5 minutes, or until the cheese is melted.

Makes one serving

SWEET AND SOUR CHICKEN

1¼ pounds boneless skinless chicken breast, cut into 1-inch cubes

1 red onion, large dice

2 green peppers, large dice

2 red peppers, large dice

½ 20-ounce can pineapple chunks in 100% pineapple juice, no sugar added
   (plus all reserved juices)

⅔ cup barbecue sauce (any brand 40 calories or less per 2 tablespoons)

2 tablespoons cider vinegar

1½ tablespoons cornstarch

3 tablespoons low-sodium soy sauce

Preheat oven to 375°F. Place the chicken, onions, and peppers in a 13 × 9 × 2-inch oven-proof baking dish. Drain the pineapple, reserving all of the juice. Add only half the drained pineapple chunks to the chicken.

In a medium saucepan, combine the reserved pineapple juice, barbecue sauce, and vinegar. Over medium heat, bring the sauce to a simmer, stirring occasionally. Meanwhile, in a small bowl, whisk together the cornstarch and soy sauce until the cornstarch is completely dissolved. Add the cornstarch mixture to the saucepan. Bring the sauce to a boil and stir until thickened, about 3 minutes. Pour the sauce over the chicken/vegetable/pineapple mixture. Cover the baking dish with aluminum foil and bake for 30 to 40 minutes, or until the chicken is no longer pink.

Makes 4 servings, 2 cups each

MARY ROSNER

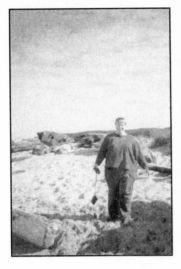 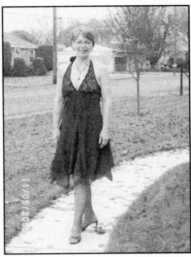

LOST: 177 pounds!

AGE: 54

HEIGHT: 5'9"

BEFORE: 345 pounds, size 28+

AFTER: 168 pounds, size 8/10

THIN ACCOMPLISHMENTS: Everything. I had to be pushed to do things, but once you accomplish one thing, you have to go find the next thing because it's a real high. Success is a real rush.

THIN CHALLENGES: None really. I love this new life.

WORDS OF WISDOM: Once you get to your goal weight, it's not like the rest of your life disappears. You can't revert to what you did before. It's not a free pass . . . it's a gift. No one can take it away, but you can choose to give it up and put your weight back on.

WHAT HAS SURPRISED YOU MOST DURING YOUR WEIGHT LOSS?

As I hit different weight-loss milestones, I saw different changes in my body. I clearly remember the first time I could tie my shoe without effort. Before, I would have to reach down, grab my pant leg (because I couldn't reach my ankle), and haul it up to my other knee so I could reach the laces. The first time I could just pick my leg up without using my hands, it shocked me.

WHAT ROLE DOES EXERCISE PLAY IN YOUR LIFE NOW?

Some of my friends think I'm a little obsessed with it, but I'm just having fun. I have two friends who also have lost a lot of weight. We go biking together, hiking, things none of us ever, ever, *ever* would have even thought of doing. I used to wonder why anyone would even want to do exercise. Now, I can't imagine my life without activity.

HOW ELSE HAS YOUR LIFE CHANGED?

The whole world has opened up. I've never done the things I'm doing now, and I'm always looking for the next grand accomplishment. Now I'm thinking maybe I want to parasail! And I've always wanted to go on a hot air balloon, but I never would have considered it when I was heavy.

ON WEIGHT-LOSS REWARDS . . .

When my daughter and I both reached our goal weights, we had a complete spa day—mud wrap, facial, massage, pedicure, manicure. Taking care of yourself is the best reward.

JOY'S LESSONS LEARNED

REWARD YOURSELF RIGHT. *Food doesn't work as a reward anymore—it isn't who you are or what you want. So what do you really want? What is your ultimate reward? Mary enjoyed head-to-toe spa pampering. But maybe you want tickets to a concert or Broadway show, a new computer or iPod, a Caribbean vacation, a tricked-out bike, or anything else that makes you feel truly and totally rewarded.*

Step Four—*Reveal* 4

s there anything quite so delicious as the taste of success? Arriving at Step Four means that you have now done what very few people are able to accomplish on their own—you have reached your goal weight. I know you can't hear it, but I'm cheering for you! Congratulations!

This is major, monumental, life-altering. Now, you can *reveal* to the world the body that has been hiding under baggy clothes and layers of fat. Even better, you can revel in your good health, energy, and optimism for the future. You can enjoy your new LIFEstyle. This is what Joy's LIFE Diet is all about—getting you to the point where you truly **Look Incredible and Feel Extraordinary**.

Once you reach your goal weight, however, you cannot go back to your old, fattening habits without regaining all those hard-lost pounds. Step Four is about helping you find your maintenance groove, a plan you can comfortably and happily live with for the rest of your life.

Eating to Maintain Weight Loss

Up till now, my LIFE Diet has been a firm guide, with food lists and rules and meal plans and recipes. I'm sure that you've learned a lot about healthy food choices and portion control, simply because you've been living with them throughout the weight-loss process. No doubt these lessons will stick with you for the rest of your life—even if you choose to ignore them.

That's the key word: choice. Maintaining weight loss is about understanding the power of choice. I have never seen a cookie jump out of a box and into someone's mouth, and that second helping of mashed potatoes doesn't accidentally fall onto a dinner plate. Those are matters of choice. You know what it took to lose weight—which means that you already know what it takes to keep it off. What makes maintenance so difficult is that you no longer have to think about *losing* weight. You are no longer "dieting." But the commitment to maintenance and good health has to be as strong as the commitment to shed pounds. Stronger, even! The fun part of losing weight is seeing your shape change in the mirror, being able to buy smaller clothes, having people tell you how wonderful you look. Now, as you move into this next phase of your life, that part of the fun is over. Now, you have to make good food choices without the immediate reward. Can you do that?

Of course you can. Your rewards go way beyond clothing and compliments. The trick is finding a way to have a healthy diet even after you no longer need to "diet." We can do that.

Step Four Rules

Step Four follows the same basic food guidelines as Step Three, however, you have more flexibility in how you choose to use your *LIFE* Extras.

Step Four Food Rules: No "Don'ts"

✓ 1. **DO** . . . weigh yourself at least once a week during Step Four.
✓ 2. **DO** . . . go back to Step One asap if the scale indicates you've gained 5 pounds.
✓ 3. **DO** . . . count all added sugar toward your daily *LIFE* Extra. (One level teaspoon sugar=16 calories and one level teaspoon of honey=20 calories! And there's three teaspoons in one tablespoon, so you can see how quickly calories add up.)
✓ 4. **DO** . . . count alcohol as a *LIFE* Extra.

✓ 5. **DO** . . . avoid trigger foods if you think they will set you off on an eating binge.

✓ 6. **DO** . . . consider carefully before adding salt to anything, but indulge moderately if you really feel you need it.

✓ 7. **DO** . . . eat all meals on a schedule and drink lots of water throughout the day.

✓ 8. **DO** . . . think about everything you eat—be conscious of your choices.

✓ 9. **DO** . . . indulge in foods on the Step Three Unlimited Foods List (on page 41–42). You can enjoy these foods in unlimited quantities at any time throughout the day, particularly when you get hungry between designated meal and snack times.

✓10. **DO** . . . feel free to swap meals or ingredients from within the same categories—choose from any of the steps.

✓11. **DO** . . . feel free to repeat a favorite meal or recipe during the week, as many times as you like (including menus from all steps).

✓12. **DO** . . . enjoy meals listed in the Step Three *LIFE* Restaurant Options when dining out (pages 202–212).

✓13. **DO** . . . feel free to substitute a frozen entrée for lunch or dinner on any night, as long as it's 350 calories or less.

✓14. **DO** . . . try making healthier versions of your personal favorite recipes (those not included in this book).

✓15. **DO** . . . feel free (if you choose) to consume up to two items each day with artificial sweetener.

✓16. **DO** . . . follow Step Four exercise guidelines.

✓17. **DO** . . . feel free to enjoy your daily 150-calorie *LIFE* Extra each day at any time you like . . . or "bank" your *LIFE* Extras.

MANDY TIDWELL

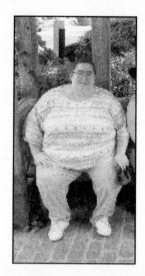

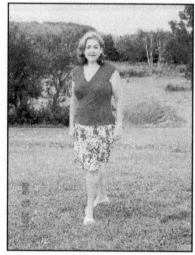

LOST: **232 pounds!**

AGE: **36**

HEIGHT: **5'4"**

BEFORE: **397 pounds, size 34+**

AFTER: **165 pounds, size 12**

THIN ACCOMPLISHMENTS: Went on a three-day backpacking trip in the Smokey Mountains. When I was hiking up a 3,500-foot mountain with a thirty-pound pack on my back, I knew that just three years ago I wouldn't have been able to get out of the car and walk across the parking lot.

THIN CHALLENGES: I know how to gain weight, and I know how to lose weight, but I have to figure out how to stay the same. I've been gaining and losing the same 5 to 10 pounds for the last year.

WORDS OF WISDOM: Set your goals and track your progress. Pick long-range and intermediate goals. And tracking reinforces that you're getting to that intermediate goal. I like making graphs and charts on the computer because I like the visual feedback.

HOW DID YOUR WEIGHT LOSS START?
I had made the decision to have weight-loss surgery, but I had to lose 25 pounds to be eligible. It seemed small enough to be achievable, whereas 200 pounds never seemed possible. Once I met that small goal, I said to myself, "Well, I did 25, let's keep going and see how far I get." I never had to have the surgery!

HOW DID YOU MAINTAIN YOUR MOTIVATION FOR MORE THAN 200 POUNDS?
I celebrated my "anniversaries" and "milestones"—every 10, 20, 50 pounds I would find some way to reward myself or share the joy. Sometimes I would just call my mom, or I would go out shopping and treat myself to a new book.

DID YOU INCLUDE EXERCISE?
I actually had a gym membership for three years before I stepped foot inside. On my first visit, I walked in and literally started with 5 minutes on the treadmill going 2 miles per hour. I gradually increased the pace and length of time. Now I'm working on jogging—and I always swore I would never jog until I saw someone who was smiling while doing it.

There is a hiking trail in Scotland called the West Highland Way. It runs 100 miles from Glasgow to Fort William. I want to do that.

JOY'S LESSONS LEARNED

SET THE GOALS YOU NEED. *Everyone is a little different—choose the* **intermediate** *and* **ultimate** *goals that make sense to you. What are your milestones? Celebrate them all! Be sure to document your impressive weight loss on a computer graph or in a journal, and review it regularly. There's nothing more motivating and encouraging than an impressive progress report!*

Banking your LIFE Extras

Step Four's challenge is to learn how your body responds to real-life eating, and to find a way to make the transition from working toward a specific goal with immediate rewards (pounds lost! clothing size falling!) to a less goal-oriented daily life where those same rewards no longer apply.

It's going to be trial and error for a while. Some weeks you'll manage everything great and feel that you'll never have to worry about food again. Other weeks may be more of a challenge. But that's how life is. Day by day, you'll figure it out. One of the easiest ways you have to tweak your diet is by choosing how you "spend" your calorie budget. The most flexible part of that budget is your daily 150-calorie *LIFE* Extra.

In Step Four, you are allowed to save up two or more days worth of these 150-calorie Extras. Here are a few scenarios you might want to consider:

+ If you're the kind of person who is methodical and you feel most comfortable when you keep your weight and eating in tight control, you'll probably want to stick with the strategy you learned in Step Three—continue to eat your daily *LIFE* Extra every day and eat sensibly all the rest of the time.

+ If you dream of eating at your favorite restaurant, then you can skip those daily *LIFE* Extras for a week and indulge that fantasy. If you don't care about bread, skip the bread basket and enjoy an entrée of your choice. But if bread is part of the allure, then go ahead and enjoy the bread, but perhaps skip the starch with dinner.

+ If you have a sweet tooth and 150 calories worth of sweets per day doesn't begin to put a dent in your desire, then skip the daily *LIFE* Extra and opt for one or two bigger desserts per week.

+ If you know that you will be attending a cocktail party, I don't want to encourage more than a drink or two. But this is real life, and I know that sometimes we plan to drink more than that. In that case, you can skip your *LIFE* Extra for a few days beforehand to save the calories (if not the hangover).

The bottom line is I don't know how your body works, so I can't give you a precise equation for what it takes for you to maintain the weight you're at now.

Some people can "fudge" a little more than others (if you'll forgive the pun), while others need to remain strictly in control. If you want to be able to enjoy flexible planning and an occasional trek to the more dangerous side of the table, I have a few last words of advice:

Watch restaurant portion sizes. In most restaurants, portions are gargantuan, especially desserts. Instead of avoiding the meal, look for ways to normalize the portions to a size you can handle. For example, many restaurants will allow you to order a half portion of some pasta or rice dishes. If the meal can't be divided, ask to have half removed from the plate and wrapped in a doggie bag before it comes to the table—that way you won't be tempted to eat it all. If all else fails and you can't safely take food home with you, leave it on the plate and walk away. Better to pay for food you didn't eat than for body fat you didn't want.

It is easier to save than to pay back. Limit the number of times you eat something outside your diet today with a promise to skip *LIFE* Extras for the next few days to make up for it. That almost never works. Invariably, another occasion or irresistible splurge will come along and your calorie debt will grow bigger and bigger, and before you know it, those splurges could show up as pounds on the scale.

"Splurge" does not mean "binge." Wild, uncontrolled eating is a binge, and that's never healthy. Even if you could bank enough calories to cover it, a binge by definition means that you are no longer in charge—you are at whim of the appetites and cravings that got you overweight in the first place. Meals should all be planned, even the splurges. You've come too far to give up what you worked so hard to attain.

And if you find the weight creeping back up, don't worry. Joy's LIFE Diet is your nutritional "home," where the door is always open. It is a strategy you can always return to if you regain weight . . . or if you simply want a refresher in healthy eating. It is your life, and your LIFE-long weight-loss plan.

Enjoying Your Success

So, what comes next?

Healthy eating is for LIFE. But that doesn't mean it has to be boring, dull, or regimented. You can discover new ways of loving food without resorting to old, unhealthy habits. With the menus and recipes throughout this book, you have the basis for a lifetime of delicious meals. Take some time to rediscover your favorite flavors, and to revive your passion for cooking by creating your own healthy masterpieces. Rediscover what it means to trust your food instincts, and to be confident in your ability to move through the world on your own, without being controlled by cravings.

But beyond that, you get the chance to redefine your life rewards. It doesn't have to be all about food. Joy Fit Club members report finding excitement and validation in new activities. Tory Klementsen has found her passion in marathons—she has run eight already and plans to run a marathon in all fifty states. Melissa Letts has been studying nutrition and hopes to be able to work with overweight teens someday. Dr. Howard Dinowitz has discovered endless energy that allows him to spend more time doing what he loves best—enjoying time with family, friends, and patients. Others have found the courage to go back to school, change jobs, change careers, write a book, learn to kayak, hike in the mountains, fly to Europe, drive across the country, and go swimming with their kids—all without fear of failure or embarrassment.

Now is the time to rediscover *your* passion. Start with the things that made you begin this journey in the first place—your family, your work, your art, your religion, your friends. You have boundless potential. With Joy's LIFE Diet, you have accomplished what most people only dream about: You have pressed the reset button on your life.

You did that!

You can do anything.

LYNN HARALDSON-BERING

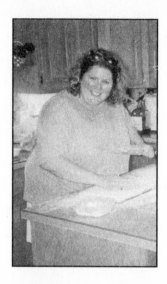

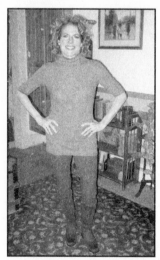

LOST: 168 pounds!

AGE: 44

HEIGHT: 5'5"

BEFORE: 296 pounds, size 30/32

AFTER: 128 pounds, size 4/6

THIN ACCOMPLISHMENTS: I went canoeing for the first time in fifteen years! I was always afraid of tipping over the boat. And I've been biking a lot, too. I love my new bike.

THIN CHALLENGES: The emotional transition to recognizing that I've reached my goal weight. I'm still trying to get comfortable with the fact that I not longer need to lose. I still check to make sure I'm not gaining, and if the scale goes up a pound, I freak out a little bit.

WORDS OF WISDOM: Losing weight is not just a diet thing—it's a mind/body/spirit thing. I had to ask myself, do I love myself enough to stay thin? Do I care enough about my future? I had to fall in love with myself a little bit, to make myself a priority and say, yeah, you are worth it.

WHAT WAS DIFFERENT ABOUT THIS ATTEMPT THAT MADE YOU SUCCESSFUL?
It was a change in mentality. If I wanted to stay thin, I had to act as though I were thin. Once I figured that out—that this is the way I'm going to be eating for the rest of my life—it was like a 2-by-4 to the head. I said to myself, I'm not going through this again. Heavy or thin, pick one. Then, accept the decision and stop bitching about it. I picked thin.

ON SPECIAL HEALTH CHALLENGES . . .
I have degenerative arthritis in most of my major joints. I need both knees replaced. My orthopedic surgeon says that my weight loss and the added muscle strength in my legs have added years to my knees. Bicycling is great, as long as I don't have to go up hills. There is an old railway that was converted by *Rails to Trails*—trains didn't run up steep hills too well, so these bike trails are wonderfully flat, safe, and easy to ride for miles. (To find one of these trails near you, search your area at *www.railstotrails.org*.)

ON THE UNEXPECTED JOYS OF WEIGHT LOSS . . .
The best part about shopping for new clothes is the underwear—the bras and panties. I was always the Granny-panty lady, but I love the pretty ones now.

JOY'S LESSONS LEARNED

IF YOU WANT TO BE THIN, THINK LIKE A THIN PERSON! *Forgo second helpings, walk instead of driving, and climb the stairs versus coasting on the escalator. Also, learn to pamper yourself with non-food rewards like an indulgent massage, a manicure/pedicure, a great haircut, a movie with friends . . . and buy new clothes. In fact, women should follow Lynn's lead and enjoy sexy lingerie! Guys can feel free to splurge on the clothing that makes them feel special—a custom-fitted suit, flat-front shorts, or (if the mood strikes) new boxers or briefs.*

Recreation—
The LIFE Exercise Program

5

Let me guess—this is the chapter you've been dreading, right? I understand. That's why I've created a program that is simple and effective and entirely do-able for everybody. Don't worry: This is going to be a breeze.

You know you need to exercise, but you probably don't do it. Only about 25 percent of all Americans engage in regular physical activity. Compare that number with this statistic from the National Weight Control Registry, which was formed to investigate what characteristics are common among people who maintained weight loss for a long time: Nearly everyone on the registry—94 percent—reported that they increased their physical activity as a way of controlling their weight. In addition, 98 percent of the registry participants changed their diets. This tells us what health experts have known all along—exercise is an important part of weight loss and maintenance, and an obvious complement to good food choices.

What's in It for Me?

Exercise has both physical and emotional benefits. Although entire books have been written about what physical activity does, here are some of the highlights:

Physically, exercise . . .

✦ *Improves blood flow.* When you walk, run, swim, bike, or do any other exercise, every inch of your body is rewarded, from your brain down to your toes. Exercise strengthens the heart so it can pump more efficiently and effectively, helps improve blood flow, ensuring that every body cell gets the oxygen and nutrients it needs for optimal performance. Exercise leads to healthier cells, which equals a healthier you. It's a whole-body experience, not just a workout for your legs.

✦ *Increases the burn.* The calorie burn, that is. Calories are units of energy that go into our body (in the form of food) and are used to keep our bodies functioning. If we eat more calories than our bodies use, then the energy is stored in the form of body fat. If we use up more calories than we eat, then our bodies take energy out of storage. Exercise requires more energy than sitting around, obviously. When you make good food choices and exercise, you will burn off more fat and lose weight.

✦ *Increases the after-burn.* Muscle uses more energy than body fat, so strengthening your muscles means you will use up more calories before, during, and after exercise. It's the nutritional equivalent of turning up your metabolic thermostat—you burn a little hotter throughout the day.

✦ *Keeps chronic diseases under control.* Exercise helps you manage heart disease by strengthening the cardiovascular system, lowering cholesterol and triglycerides, and improving blood pressure. It also improves control over insulin levels of type 2 diabetes, keeps bowels regular, and contributes to bone strength. Exercise also reduces the pain of arthritis. Cancer survivors are encouraged to exercise as a way of improving immunity.

✦ *Tones muscles.* Muscle is more compact than fat; it takes up less space. When you exercise, your muscles become firmer and tighter, not big and bulky. Think of where the largest muscles are in your body—your thighs, butt, midsection (the abs), back, and chest. Would you like them to be firmer and tighter? If you said yes, exercise is the only way to do that.

So to summarize, the benefits of daily low-impact cardiovascular exercise are:

+ Improves the functioning of the cardiovascular system
+ Increases good cholesterol (HDLs)
+ Improves blood flow
+ Reduces the risk of cardiovascular disease
+ Helps burn fat and calories
+ Helps increase metabolism
+ Improves energy levels
+ Strengthens bones, muscles, ligaments, tendons, and cartilage
+ Combats chronic diseases such as type 2 diabetes, osteoporosis, and certain types of cancer

Not impressed yet?

Emotionally, exercise . . .

+ *Makes you happier.* Exercise helps the body create and release brain chemicals that can improve your mood and make you feel calmer and less stressed.
+ *Makes you feel empowered.* Those same brain chemicals that make you happy also combat depression and anxiety, leaving you less worried and fretful. And when you end up with a fit, toned body, you will naturally feel more confident. Overall, exercise is the biggest ego-booster out there. Plus, it all builds! If you feel better about yourself, you'll want to take care of yourself, so staying healthy by eating right and exercising will become second nature.
+ *Improves memory.* In order to function properly, brain cells need even more oxygen and nutrients than other body cells. A sluggish brain can cause you to be more forgetful. Exercise won't give you a flawless memory, just a better one.
+ *Improves your relationships.* A friend told me that she and her husband walk two miles around their neighborhood every night. It started as a way to exercise together, but it has become much more. Every day they have a

solid half hour to do nothing but talk with each other, sometimes about important events, but most of the time about small observations and feelings. My friend is convinced that these nightly walks and conversations have made them closer, and is part of the reason their marriage has lasted twenty-five years. Grab your significant other or a friend you'd like to know better and walk together.

SISSY LUSK

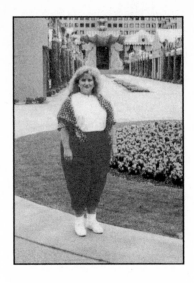 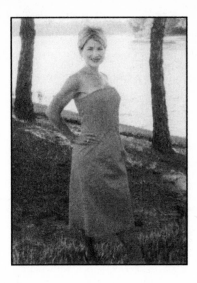

LOST: **215 pounds!**

AGE: **43**

HEIGHT: **5'2"**

BEFORE: **345 pounds, size "the largest I could find"**

AFTER: **130 pounds, size 4/6**

THIN ACCOMPLISHMENTS: **My biggest accomplishment is keeping the weight off, of course. But I'm also pretty proud of having gone on a 30-mile bike ride with my husband.**

THIN CHALLENGES: **My biggest challenge is keeping exercise going. I used to exercise five days a week, and took weekends off. But it was so hard to get started again on Monday that I found it easier to exercise every day of the week.**

WORDS OF WISDOM: **Every single pound you lose is a success! Making your goal weight is great, but I think every little step along the way is a reason to be proud.**

WHAT MADE YOU DECIDE TO TRY TO LOSE WEIGHT THIS TIME?

I went to pay for gas in a convenience store. It was crowded with construction work-ers, and behind me was a mom and her little boy. He asked me why I was so fat. I tried to ignore him, but the mom made the little guy apologize. With everyone watching, he pitched a fit, but grudgingly said, "I'm sorry I said you were fat." When I got back to my car, I sat there and just cried. I started the diet that night. That mother and son don't know it, but I thank them for saving my life. It was painful, but it was my wake-up call.

WHAT DO YOU THINK MADE YOU SUCCESSFUL THIS TIME AROUND?

This time, time didn't matter. I didn't let myself get overwhelmed. However long it took, I was going to see it through.

DID EXERCISE PLAY A PART?

Definitely. At first, I was intimidated by the gym. I walked by and looked in the win-dow just to see what type of people were in there. Most of them looked like me. At first, they tried to talk me out of the yearly membership. They didn't think I would keep at it. That stayed in the back of my mind. All year long, I kept saying to myself, "Don't you dare quit because it will show that they were right."

ON FIGHTING FOR SUCCESS . . .

Make a list of other things you've achieved that took work—graduating college, paying off a credit card. You had the strength to succeed then, now put those same strengths into losing weight. Concentrate on your successes, not your failures.

JOY'S LESSONS LEARNED

LOSING WEIGHT IS NOT A RACE. *The time will pass anyway. Two years from now, would you rather be the person you are today, or a thinner ver-sion of you?*

Yeah, but . . .

Before getting to the nitty-gritty of the program, I think it is important to acknowledge that some people hate exercise. I think that's because they simply haven't found the right activity, or they haven't been properly introduced to the concept of exercise as recreation. Isn't that a great word? *Recreation* has a double meaning: 1—something done for fun; and 2—the act of making or creating something all over again. Exercise really does offer a way for us to remake or remodel our bodies! So why do so many of us avoid activities that might cause us to break a sweat?

Fight or Flight? Most Pick Flight

Think of a time when you experienced free and easy movement. What comes to mind? Most people come up with a memory from their childhood—running down a grassy hill or on the playground, dancing like a rock star in their bedrooms, playing soccer, jumping rope, climbing and swinging off just about anything. Movement was fun! Then we got to gym class where we were rated, graded, and compared. While some people thrive in that kind of environment, others fade. What used to be fun became stressful. And because all living things naturally avoid things that cause stress—that famous *fight-or-flight* instinct—it really isn't surprising that so many of us hear the word "exercise" and run the other way (not literally, of course—that would be exercise). There are a few things you can do to put your mind in a more exercise-friendly state.

✦ *Choose to "fight" instead of flee.* If the brain's choice is fight or flight, enlist your competitive instinct and join the battle. For example, you can set goals and try to beat them, or hold a friendly competition with an exercise buddy, or even decide not to let a little activity be the thing that beats you. Joy Fit Club member Sissy Lusk fought back when her gym tried to sell her a more expensive month-to-month membership instead of the full-year option. They didn't think she would last longer than a month. Sissy took the dare, bought the full-year membership, and whenever she felt like dropping out she remembered that she didn't want to let them be the ones to say "I told you so."

✦ *Make exercise the lesser of two evils.* For several of members of my Fit Club, exercise only became a regular part of their lives after they experienced a serious health threat. Then, walking was a whole lot less stressful than the risk of a heart attack. Others weighed the stress of exercise against the stress of not being able to play with their grandchildren. Put in context of your whole life, exercise is not that bad. If you find an outcome that motivates you, hold onto it.

✦ *Make exercise less stressful.* You can change the rules of the fight-or-flight response by taking away the "stress" part of the equation and by adding positive elements that make exercise more enjoyable. In the beginning, that might mean pairing exercise with something you love. If you are a shopaholic, you might try mall-walking—as long as you don't drift into a store before your minutes are up! A lot of my clients find that the buddy system—teaming up with a person or group for regular exercise sessions—helps keep everyone motivated. In a time when we all find it difficult to keep in touch with friends, walking with a buddy, either in person or on a hands-free phone, can be a real gift.

One of the best ideas I've heard recently is to take discussion clubs on the road. Book clubs are notorious for being glorified excuses for drinking wine and eating cookies while flopped on a couch. Why not put on some walking shoes and take the club outside, away from food, alcohol, and extra pounds? One woman told me that she and her husband have a book club of their own. They listen to the audio books . . . *but they can only listen while they are exercising!* They look forward to exercising because they get involved in the books and want to hear the endings. I can't help but imagine the possibilities of this type of incentive. Imagine if teenagers could only talk on the phone while on a treadmill, or if kids could only listen to music while cleaning their rooms. Fabulous!

✦ *Stop calling it "exercise."* For some people, that word is so loaded with negative images and emotions they can't get past it. Try giving "exercise" a mental make-over. Instead of saying you are going out to *exercise*, say you are going out for *some private time*, or *play time*, or that you are *reenergizing*. Use anything that works to trick your mind into supporting your new level of activity.

✦ *Join the club—or at least join the others!* You may find it a lot easier to stick with a program if you know there are hundreds or thousands of other people facing the same challenges. Consider joining the online program at www.JoyBauer.com, where you can form real friendships with real people in a virtual location. It helps!

Not a Minute to Spare

Lack of time to exercise is by far the most common excuse I hear. When your day already feels packed from the minute you get up to the moment you lie down in bed, exercise can feel impossible. Really, "lack of time" is another way of saying "I don't want to exercise." We all seem to find time to do things we want to do during the day—shop, watch television or YouTube, search the Internet for random information, play video games, anything. If you really wanted to exercise, you would find time to do it. Some of the busiest people I know manage to fit quite a lot of physical activity into their days. You may need to rearrange your schedule a bit, but the time is there.

Imagine it like this: Let's say you're on a strict monetary budget, with not a nickel to spare. If you then discover that your child needs orthodontic braces, you'd find the money for them. What if someone offered you a two-week vacation in Hawaii, all expenses paid except for meals—would you find a way to take the trip? Sure you would. Money might be tight, but there's usually a way to cut the budget in some areas to pay for things that are really needed or desperately wanted. The same goes for time. Think of exercise as one of those necessary "expenses."

TAMMY STEPHENSON

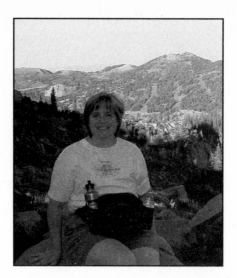 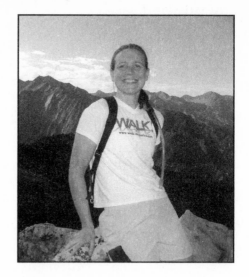

LOST: **105 pounds!**

AGE: **37**

HEIGHT: **5'8"**

BEFORE: **250 pounds, size 24**

AFTER: **145 pounds, size 6**

THIN ACCOMPLISHMENTS: I've done three half-marathons, and I'm going to do a full marathon this fall. This summer, I'm going to enter the USA Track and Field Masters National Championship race walk.

THIN CHALLENGES: Emotional eating. I struggle with eating when I feel a little down, thinking it will make me feel better. But I know that it might make me feel better for ten minutes, and then I'll feel even worse because I ate too much.

WORDS OF WISDOM: If you're an emotional eater, you need to figure out other things to fill your emotional needs—call a friend, read a book, have a hot cup of tea, curl up in a warm blanket. Figure out what you're trying to get from the food and look for a way to get that feeling a different way.

I was motivated by the birth of my first child. I didn't want him to grow up and learn the same lousy eating habits I had. I was a slave to food; I didn't want that for my son.

SO YOUR WEIGHT LOSS WAS ALL AS AN EXAMPLE FOR HIM?

That was a big part of it, but I knew, too, that I was unhappy as a fat person. I ate for emotional reasons; it made me feel good to eat. I came to a point when I realized food wasn't my friend; it was making my life miserable.

ON FEELING GUILTY . . .

I always felt guilty about what I was eating. The first week on my diet, I didn't feel guilty anymore because I knew I was eating "properly." I knew that I needed to do this for the rest of my life, and that was going to be okay.

ON BECOMING ACTIVE . . .

I was a lifetime couch potato. Exercise has become very important to me, and that's quite unexpected. I tried a few different things before deciding that race walking is my "thing." For anyone who thinks she hates exercise, I say keep searching until you find one you love.

JOY'S LESSONS LEARNED

FIND NEW OUTLETS FOR YOUR EMOTIONS. *Emotional eating is very common in times of stress, anxiety, sadness, and most other emotions. The trick is to spend less time fixated on food by redirecting your focus and energy. Tammy discovered a passion for race walking, but there is a world of activity that can busy your hands and mind, including quilting, sewing, volunteer work, dancing, taking classes, playing cards, reading, gardening, woodworking, writing, painting, etc.*

LIFE Exercise Steps

Step One: Release (one week)

GOAL: *To take off excess "bloat."*

YOUR COMMITMENT: *30 to 60 minutes of some kind of low-impact cardiovascular exercise—walking is recommended—every single day for 7 days without exception.*

In Step One, you have the option to do your workouts in Full Portions or Bite-Sized Pieces.

+ *Full Portion Exercise*—Do your entire daily workout in a single session totaling between 30 and 60 minutes. For example, you might walk outdoors for 30 minutes before work; or perhaps you might hit the gym for 45 minutes before dinner.

  Full Portion Exercise is the best option for most people. If your schedule permits, the ideal way to stay committed to a regular exercise program is to get it out of the way first thing in the morning. As the day goes on, more and more things have the potential to pop up, interrupt your schedule, and thwart your workout plans. The beauty of exercising in the morning is that typically there are fewer distractions so you can do it all, be done with it, and then go about your day. In fact, studies show that morning exercisers are 50 percent more likely to stick with their program than those who exercise at other times of day.

+ *Bite-Sized Pieces*—Do several smaller exercise sessions spaced throughout the day, but still adding up to a total of 30 to 60 minutes. For example, you could take a brisk 10-minute walk with the dog in the morning, another 10-minute walk at midday on your lunch break, and another 10-minute walk after dinner with a friend.

  The Bite-Sized Pieces option works well for those who are challenged to find 30 to 60 minutes they can set aside for exercise each day. This exercise

WHAT IS "LOW-IMPACT CARDIOVASCULAR EXERCISE"?

Low-impact exercise is any fitness activity where one foot is completely on the ground (or in contact with the exercise machine) at all times. For example, walking is low-impact, but running is high-impact.

Cardiovascular exercise is sustained, rhythmic, full-body movements that raise heart rate. The more you move your body, the more your body demands oxygen, which means that the higher the intensity of the exercise, the greater number of calories you'll burn.

In Step One, you are just beginning to establish the habit of regular daily exercise to burn calories and speed fat loss. By keeping the activities low-impact, you'll protect your joints, muscles, and tendons from overuse injuries. Walking is the easiest choice because it is accessible to pretty much everyone. You don't need a treadmill—just walk out of your door and time yourself for a minimum of 15 minutes in one direction. Then turn around and head back home. It's as simple as that.

Other low-impact exercises include biking outdoors, stationary biking, elliptical machines, stair climbing machines, cross-country skiing, step aerobics, low-impact aerobics, cardio kickboxing, water aerobics, and swimming.

schedule works best for those with demanding full-time jobs, and also for moms with young children. For those who are very out of shape, doing exercise in Bite-Sized Pieces allows them to take recovery breaks between spurts of exercise.

Another bonus of this workout schedule is that some studies suggest that this type of "intermittent" exercise, broken into separate segments, may raise metabolism higher and for a longer period of time after the workout than workouts done all in one shot.

WHY CAN'T I JUST START RUNNING?

Many people believe that running is the best way to get in shape. While it is true that running is an excellent fitness activity, it is only appropriate for a select few individuals because it places a great deal of stress on the muscles, tendons, and joints. When you run, your feet hit the ground with a force 2½ to 3 times your body weight. So for example if you weigh 160 lbs, you hit the ground with a force of 400 to 480 lbs. It's not surprising that runners are far more likely than walkers to be injured. The more you run, the greater your risk of injury. Walking, on the other hand, is not associated with increased risk of injury.

Running is an activity best reserved for the very fit, and those with smaller frames and lower body weight. Think about it: How many guys who look like they shop in the Big and Tall Men's section are running in the front of the pack at the New York City Marathon?

Walking Guidelines

Walking for fitness is a little different from the way you walk throughout the rest of your day. To get the most out of your daily exercise, keep these guidelines in mind:

1. *Walk with Intensity.* You want to feel that your walk is challenging, but not exhausting. I love to recommend the "talk test" as a way to tell if you are exercising at the proper intensity—you should be able to talk without gasping for air, but not have so much breath that you can sing. If you walk with a buddy, you can watch out for each other, slowing down if you hear signs that the walk is too intense, or picking up the pace if the talk comes too easily. (And yes, you can try singing a few notes to test your intensity. After a while, the right pace will become second nature.)

   Alternatively, if you like gadgets, you can use your heart rate as an intensity guide. A heart rate monitor is a worthwhile investment, because it does this for you and can motivate you to challenge yourself.

ABOUT HEART RATE MONITORS

A heart rate monitor is a device that measures and monitors your heart rate. It takes the guesswork out of figuring out whether you are walking at a sufficient intensity to improve fitness, and it can motivate you to stay on track with your program. In fact, many models act as virtual coaches, tracking your daily workouts and letting you know if you've met your weekly goals.

A heart rate monitor typically consists of a wrist unit (like a watch with additional functions) and a transmitter strap with electrodes attached to your chest. Before your workout, the monitor will need to be programmed with information about your age and gender, and, depending on the model you choose, perhaps also your height, weight, how often you work out, and your current fitness level. The unit will calculate your heart rate training zone from the information that you enter. Then, as you walk or run, the monitor will give you feedback about how your heart rate compares with your goal so you know whether to speed up, slow down, or keep moving at the same pace.

If you are intimidated by anything technical, then you can certainly use the "talk test" instead of worrying about electrodes and programming. But if you're a technophile, you'll probably be fascinated by the many features available on some of the high-end heart rate monitors, which include the ability to load your workouts onto a home computer, specialized data analysis software, and the ability to customize programs in different heart rate intensity training zones.

2. *Focus on Fast Feet.* When challenged to walk faster, many people make the mistake of taking bigger strides. With fitness walking, the idea is to take a normal stride—step length—the same as you would during a typical daily

walk, but to "turn them over" faster. Imagine that a large hand is pushing you along from behind, urging you to go faster. (If you're a mom or dad, you may have done this with your own kids!)

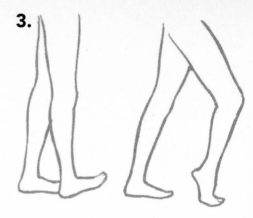

3. *Roll through Your Whole Foot.* This advice may sound a little crazy, but you would be surprised at how many people plod flat-footed. Women who love to wear stilettos can develop foot-placement habits that are great for balancing on heels, but are exactly the reverse of the foot placement needed for fitness walking. As you walk, the first part of your foot that should hit pavement is the heel. Then, roll through the entire foot and push off with the toe. Depending on your personal walking habits, this may not feel "natural" to you. For the first few sessions, you may need to concentrate on this pattern

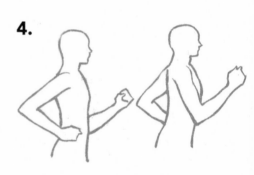

with every step—hit with the heel, roll through the entire foot, push off with the toe. Although thinking about each step may slow you down at the beginning, you will eventually be walking in relative hyper-speed.

4. *Use Power Arms.* Effective fitness walking involves your whole body, including your upper torso and arms. "Power Arms" don't just swing at your side; they are purposeful and active. Power Arms automatically make your feet move faster, which raises your heart rate and helps you burn more fat and calories. To use Power Arms:

✦ Begin by making little fists with your hands. Don't squeeze, just close them loosely, as if you were holding a small bird that you didn't want to hurt, but you didn't want to fly away. (If you are one of those people who tend to tense up, carry foam balls or loose balls of aluminum foil, and try not to compact them as you walk.)

5.

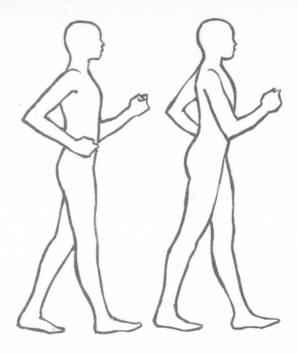

♦ Keeping your arms in close toward your body, bend your elbows at a 90 degree angle.

♦ As you walk, your arms will develop a natural swing. Once you have the rhythm, concentrate on driving your elbows back, keeping the fists closed and the arms in close to the sides of your body.

♦ As you walk, think to yourself "drive, drive, drive," as you continually pump your arms, driving your elbows back behind you.

5. *Maintain Good Posture.* If you thought the days of being nagged by someone to "stand up straight" ended when you left home, think again! Good posture is about more than how you look, it's about helping your body move as efficiently as possible, while also strengthening your core and protecting your spine. When you walk (or stand or sit, for that matter) with good posture, you activate your abdominals, which trains your core. To maintain good posture while walking:

♦ Imagine the top of your head reaching toward the sky (or ceiling). Your chin should be parallel to the horizon, your nose and eyes pointed forward.

+ Think about lifting your chest while keeping your shoulders back and down. Imagine that you are trying to measure an inch taller, with no hunching or drooping.

+ Think also about holding your midsection solid as if you were getting ready for someone to punch you in the stomach. This activates the abdominals and lower back muscles, which not only keeps your core stable, it also lets you generate more power with your arms and legs.

step one exercise

Monday	Tuesday	Wednesday	Thursday	Friday	Saturday	Sunday
30-60 min	30-60 min	30-60 min	30-60 min	30-60 min	30-60 min	30-60 min
Cardio	Cardio	Cardio	Cardio	Cardio	Cardio	Cardio

in a nutshell

Step Two: Relearn (2 weeks)

GOAL: *To relearn how to move your body and make fitness a part of your life*

YOUR COMMITMENT:

+ *7 days per week do 30 to 60 minutes of walking or other low-impact cardiovascular exercise; 3 days per week add Speed Play*
+ *3 to 5 days per week do LIFE Enhancers*

The Step Two exercises are very exciting because they add a *LIFE* Enhancers workout—a 5 to 10 minute series of poses and stretches that help to eliminate some of the most common pain and stiffness problems many people experience. Back pain? Leg aches? Shoulder stiffness? *LIFE* Enhancers can fix that! What could be simpler? I think you are going to love this step.

Walking Guidelines

The goal of Step Two is to continue to walk (or do other cardiovascular exercise) a minimum of 30 minutes every day. I realize that life sometimes intervenes and walking might be difficult or impossible on a particular day. If you miss a day or two, I don't want you to stress about it. Although seven days a week is optimal, five days a week is good. But one of the main goals of the entire LIFE exercise program is to make movement a part of your everyday lifestyle. I want you to awaken every morning with a little mental sticky note reminding you to get up and get moving.

Just as in Step One, you can complete your walk continuously in one Full Portion, or break the time up into Bite-Sized Pieces throughout the day. Keep in mind your intensity, posture, power arms, and fast feet.

Step Two introduces a fun twist on the plain old walk. On three out of your seven days of walking, I want you to practice a form of "Speed Play." Every so often during your walk, imagine that your sneakers have booster rockets on them, turn on the boosters and ramp up your speed for a few minutes. You make the rules of this game. You can target a particular mailbox or light post in the distance and speed up until you reach that point. Then, return to your usual pace. Do this several times during the walk . . . and put equal emphasis on "speed" and "play." Make it fun with mini challenges for yourself. Every time you turn on those booster rockets, you'll be burning more calories and helping your weight drop off more quickly.

LIFE Enhancers

These fabulous exercises are deceptively simple. After the first day, when you'll be learning the *LIFE* Enhancers, going through the whole routine should take no longer than five to ten minutes. You can do these exercises before or after your continuous walks, or separately. Just put on clothing that allows you to move, claim a space on a carpeted floor or mat, and work through these poses.

Note: while performing these exercises, be strong but gentle. Do not bully your way through, and try not to become frustrated if these simple exercises end up to be more difficult `than you thought. Do what you can—your strength and endurance will improve quickly. If you love these Enhancers and want to add more to your routine, go to www.JoyBauer.com.

1. BIRD DOG

Strengthens core, reduces back pain

✦ Get on all fours with your hands directly underneath your shoulders and your knees directly underneath your hips. Flatten your back like a tabletop.

✦ Keeping your back flat and your hips level, extend your right arm forward and your left leg back so that they are parallel to the floor, in a straight line with your back. Keep your abdominals solid as if you were bracing yourself against a punch in the stomach. Hold this position for a 3 second count, then lower to the starting position.

✦ Do 8 on one side, and then switch and do 8 on the other side. Do a total of 2 sets per side.

1.

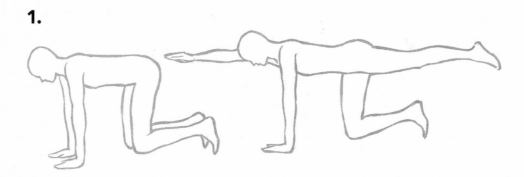

2. PELVIC BRIDGES

Strengthens core, increases mobility in hips, tones buttocks

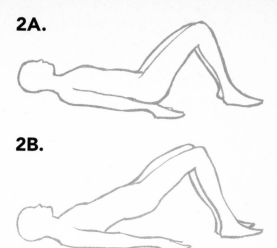

2A.

2B.

+ Lie flat on your back with your knees bent, feet flat on the floor.
+ Squeeze your buttocks and lift your pelvis up off of the floor as high as you can without straining. Hold the squeeze at the top for a 3 second count, then slowly lower down to starting position.
+ Do 2 sets of 12 repetitions.

3. DEAD BUGS

Strengthens core

+ Lie flat on your back with your knees bent at a 90 degree angle, feet off the floor. Reach with your hands up as if you were trying to push the ceiling away from you.
+ Tighten up your core as if you were bracing to get a punch to your gut. Press your back down into floor and try not to move your torso.
+ Simultaneously lower your left arm back over your head, and your right leg down and away until both are parallel with the floor. Slowly return to the starting position and switch to the other arm and leg.
+ Continue alternating between left arm/right leg and right arm/left leg, keeping your torso still throughout. Do 2 sets of these alternating repetitions, 16–20 repetitions per set.

3A.   **3B.**

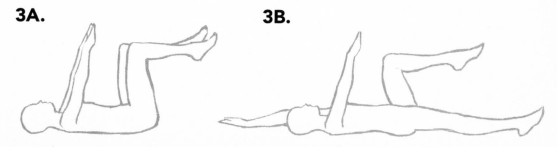

4. WALKING INTO WALLS
Stretches calf muscles

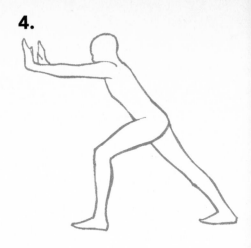

✦ Stand two to three feet from a wall. Place your hands on the wall in a "push-up type" position. Step forward with one foot until it is about 18 inches away from the wall.

✦ Lean forward into the wall with your arms, keeping the heel of your back foot on the floor. You should feel a strong stretch in the calf of the back leg.

✦ Hold for the stretch for 30 seconds to a minute. Repeat 2 times on each leg.

5. DOORWAY STRETCH
Stretches chest and shoulders

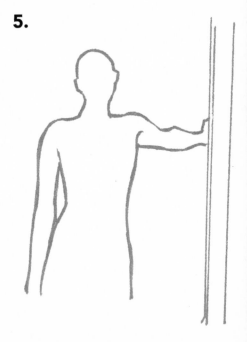

✦ Stand in doorway and place your right hand on the inside of the doorway with your thumb up. The arm should be chest height.

✦ Step forward 2 feet with your left leg until you feel a stretch in the front of the right shoulder and the right side of your chest.

✦ Hold the stretch for 30 seconds to a minute. Repeat 2 times on each side.

6. NECK STRETCHES
Stretches the neck

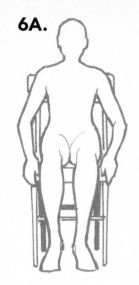
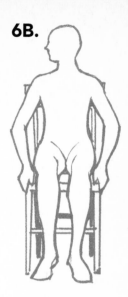

6A. **6B.**

- ✦ Sit upright in a chair with good posture.
- ✦ Look over your right shoulder as far as you can, hold for a second. Return to center. Then look over your left shoulder as far as you can, hold for a second. Repeat 6 times on each side.
- ✦ Maintaining good posture, lower your left ear toward your left shoulder. Hold the stretch for 30 seconds to a minute. Switch to other side, lowering right ear toward your right shoulder. Repeat twice for each side.

7. COBRA STRETCH
Stretches core and realigns spine

- ✦ Lie face down, elbows bent, arms close to your body with your forearms on the floor.
- ✦ Squeeze your buttocks, press your pelvis down into the floor, and gently press up so that your upper torso, shoulders, and head are off the floor. You should feel a gentle stretch in the front of your body. You should not feel any pinching or discomfort in your lower back.
- ✦ Hold the stretch for 30 seconds to a minute. Repeat 2 times.

7.

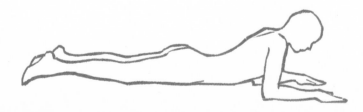

step two exercise

Monday	Tuesday	Wednesday	Thursday	Friday	Saturday	Sunday
30-60 min	30-60 min	30-60 min	30-60 min	30-60 min	30-60 min	30-60 min
Cardio	Cardio	Cardio	Cardio	Cardio	Cardio	Cardio
With	+	With	+	With	+	
Speed Play	Life	Speed Play	Life	Speed Play	Life	
	Enchancers		Enchancers		Enchancers	

in a nutshell

(This is an example of a typical week.
You may add Speed Play and LIFE Enhancers to any day you wish.
Speed Play should not be done two days in a row.)

Step Three: Reshape (until goal weight is reached)

GOAL: *To reshape, tighten, and tone your body with fat-burning cardio, and sculpt shapely, sexy muscles with resistance training*

YOUR COMMITMENT:

+ *5 to 7 days per week do 30 to 60 minutes of walking or other low-impact cardiovascular exercise. 2 to 3 days per week add Speed Play to your walk*
+ *2 days per week do LIFE Enhancers (from Step Two) and Resistance Training*

In Step One, you jumped in with both feet to make a commitment to regular daily exercise. In Step Two you learned how to ramp up the intensity of your cardiovascular workouts with Speed Play bursts to make them more effective. Now in Step Three, it's time to add in another critical piece of the fat loss equation: resistance training.

What is resistance training?

Resistance training is the process of using weights, specialized bands, machines, even your own body weight to improve muscular fitness, including both strength (how much weight you can lift) and muscular endurance (how many times you can lift a given weight without muscle fatigue). The body's muscles pull or push against a weight or other form of resistance, forcing them to work harder.

Resistance training is a key component of any well-rounded weight loss program. This is because when we lose weight we not only lose body fat, we lose lean body tissue as well. This is problematic because loss of lean body tissue means a lower metabolic rate, which means that it is more difficult to lose weight or maintain weight loss . . . and it also becomes easier to gain weight in the future.

There are many different techniques using different kinds of equipment, such as free weights, hand weights, circuit training, and resistance bands. The program here is a simple, beginner-level group of exercises. Some require hand weights, but most use your own body weight as a resistance. If you have a light set of dumbbells—2-, 3-, or 4-pound weights—they will come in handy. If not, you can use unopened cans of soup (or cans of anything else, about 16 ounces) or create your own weights using water in quart-sized milk jugs (the kind with handles). You may want to find a good workout mat if you will be working on a hard floor. On carpeting, you can simply lay down a large bath towel to keep fibers off of you . . . and to keep sweat off the rug!

The Step Three Circuit Workout

This resistance workout is in the form of a circuit. It is a series of exercises designed to be completed one right after another in a precise order. There is no waiting between exercises.

Circuit workouts burn more calories *during* the workout because you are continuously moving the largest muscle groups in a rhythmic fashion, and *after* the workout because they are more intense, which means that you continue to burn extra calories even *after* you've stopped exercising. Perhaps best of all, circuit workouts are time efficient, making it easier to do your routine and get on with your day. This circuit has been specially designed to provide a beginner with a quick (but still balanced) workout for your entire body.

The Step Three Circuit Workout can be done on the same day as your cardio-vascular exercise, or on a different day. Doing it after continuous cardio is help-ful because walking will get your body warm and prepare your muscles and joints for resistance training. This option is best if you have a larger block of time you can devote to fitness. If you choose to do the Circuit Workout alone (without cardio first), take 3 to 5 minutes to march in place before beginning to warm-up.

Before beginning the circuit, do the *LIFE* Enhancers workout (from Step 2). Then, perform one set of all six exercises in the order presented. When you've fin-ished the whole circuit, take a 3 to 5 minute break, then complete a second set. That's the whole secret to a stronger you!

(If you enjoy this workout and want to get additional exercise variations or go a step or two further, visit my website at www.JoyBauer.com.)

RESISTANCE TRAINING TIPS

- Don't do resistance training two days in a row—always be sure to leave a day in between to give your body a chance to repair and recover.
- Do not hold your breath during the workout. Breathe deeply in through your nose and out through your mouth.
- If you become nauseous or dizzy, stop and take a break. Return when/if you feel able.
- Be patient with yourself. You may not be able to do the entire 30 seconds the first few times that you do the workouts. Be consist-ent and soon you will find that you are able to do more and more with less effort.

How to Do the *LIFE* Step Three Circuits

- ✦ Warm up with 3 to 5 minutes of walking, dancing, or other full-body movement.
- ✦ Then, do 2 sets of each of the *LIFE* Enhancers exercises from Step 1 as a warm up.
- ✦ Then, do all 6 exercises of the circuit *in order*. Do each exercise for 30 seconds, using a moderate tempo—don't rush through, but don't dawdle, either. When you have finished all the exercises, rest for 3 to 5 minutes, then do all six again.

1. SUMO SQUATS

Works the hips, buttocks, and inner thighs

- ✦ Stand with your legs about 2 feet apart.
- ✦ Place your hands on your hips and, keeping your torso upright, bend your knees and lower your tailbone straight down to the floor. Go down only as far as you feel comfortable.
- ✦ Then straighten your legs and return to the starting position. Continue for 30 seconds.

1.

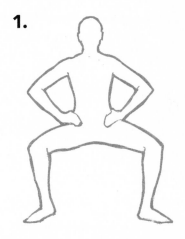

2. ALTERNATING BACK LUNGES

Works the hips, thighs, and buttocks

- ✦ Stand tall with your hands on your hips.
- ✦ In one smooth motion, step back with your *right* leg and lower your right knee toward the ground, without actually touching the knee to the ground.

2A. **2B.**

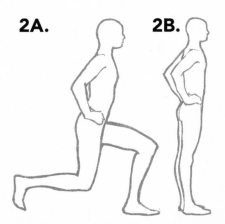

- ✦ Return to the starting position, and repeat the movement with the *left* leg.
- ✦ Continue, alternating legs, for 30 seconds.

3. SIDE-TO-SIDE LUNGES
Works the inner and outer thighs

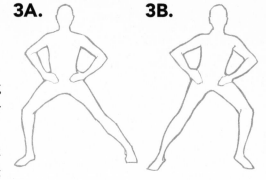

3A. **3B.**

- ✦ Stand tall with your feet a few inches apart.
- ✦ Step out about 2 feet to your *right*, bending your *right* knee and sitting back with your buttocks.
- ✦ Return to the center and then step out about 2 feet to your *left*, bending your *left* knee and sitting back with your buttocks.
- ✦ Continue, alternating sides, for 30 seconds.

4. MODIFIED PUSH-UPS
Works the chest, shoulders, and triceps

- ✦ Get on your knees in a push-up position. Your hands should be in line with the center of your chest, below your shoulders, fingers facing forward.
- ✦ Press your body up, keeping your torso still and abdominals drawn in tight.
- ✦ Try to continue for 30 seconds. If this is too difficult, you can do your push-ups from a standing position with your hands on a wall. If it is too easy, you can do the push-ups on your toes instead of your knees.

4A. **4B.**

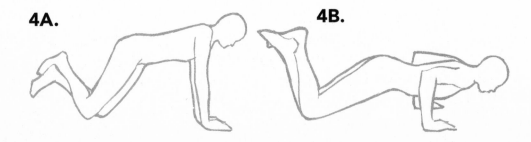

5. SEATED ROWS
Works the back, back of the shoulders, and biceps

✦ Sit on the edge of a chair (one without arms). Place a rolled up towel or small pillow in your lap for support, lean forward, and rest your chest on it. Your back should be flat at a 45-degree angle.

✦ Hold the lightest weight dumbbells (or a soup can) in your hands. Let your arms hang down by the side of your body.

✦ With your arms close to your side, bend your elbows and pull them backward, keeping your shoulders down and squeezing the muscles in between your shoulder blades. The motion should approximate rowing or starting a lawnmower with a pull-cord.

✦ Lower your arms, and repeat. Continue for 30 seconds.

5A.

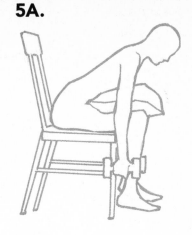

5B.

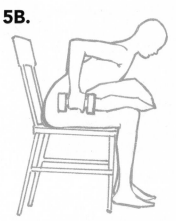

6. SEATED REVERSE FLY
Works the middle of the back

✦ Sit on the edge of a chair (one without arms). Place a rolled up towel or small pillow in your lap for support, lean forward, and rest your chest on it. Your back should be flat at a 45-degree angle.

✦ Hold the lightest weight dumbbells (or soup can) in your hands. Keeping your elbows straight, let your arms hang down by the side of your body.

✦ Keeping your shoulders down, squeeze the muscles in between your shoulder blades and raise your arms until they are parallel with the floor.

✦ Lower your arms, and repeat. Continue for 30 seconds.

6A.

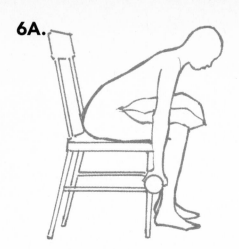

6B.

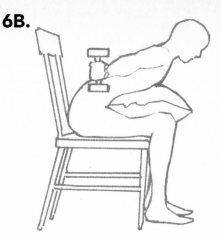

step three exercise

Monday	Tuesday	Wednesday	Thursday	Friday	Saturday	Sunday
30-60 min	30-60 min	Life	30-60 min	30-60 min	Life	30-60 min
Cardio	Cardio	Enhancers	Cardio	Cardio	Enhancers	Cardio
	with	+	with		+	with
	Speed Play	Resistance	Speed Play		Resistance	Speed Play
		Training			Training	

in a nutshell

(This is an example of a typical week.
Cardio is required 5 days per week; 7 days per week is optional.
Use Speed Play with any cardio day, but not two days in a row.
Add resistance training 2 days per week, leaving a minimum of one day in between.
LIFE Enhancers may be done all 7 days per week. Remember, you can get a customized workout plan by joining the
online program at www.JoyBauer.com.)

Step Four: Reveal (Maintenance)

GOAL: *To reveal the new you, and keep weight from coming back*

YOUR COMMITMENT: *To adopt a lifestyle that includes movement!*

My guess is that you've gotten a pretty good workout just jumping up and down with happiness at reaching your goal weight. That's a great start . . . but let's take it further.

If you have been following the exercise portion of my LIFE Diet, then you know the benefits of exercise. You may not always have enjoyed it, but you can't argue with the results. Today, you are probably healthier, thinner, fitter, and have more energy than ever before. Now I want you to take that energy out into the world and do something *fun*.

The goal for Step Four is to find activities you enjoy that do not revolve around food. Maybe you discovered that you really enjoy walking in the early mornings before the roads get crowded, or maybe you've discovered your inner Arnold Schwarzenegger and want to get deeper into resistance training—that's great. By all means continue walking and lifting. But you are not limited to these few exercises. There are so many exciting activities out there that I'm sure something will call out to you. All help burn calories, keep weight down, and keep your muscles toned and fit (see chart).

Physically, you are a different person today than you were just a few months ago. Maybe you didn't think you could ever climb a mountain, but maybe you can now. You'll never know until you try. Maybe you were too self-conscious to try salsa or belly dancing, water polo, squash, or yoga, but maybe your perspective has changed. Give it a shot. Many of my Fit Club members told me that one of their greatest joys was fulfilling a dream of being able to go canoeing or kayaking. Because of their size, they hadn't even been able to step on a floating dock before, and they worried about capsizing the boat. Once they lost their weight, they became avid water sports fans. Their size had been holding them back from doing the things they loved.

It's time to rediscover the joys of active recreation. Which activities have been missing from your life? What dreams have been out of your reach? Try them again. You may be surprised at all you can do.

MOVE IT . . . AND LOSE IT

Calorie Burning Chart by Activity

(approximate calories burned per hour
based on 150 lb person)

Golf, with cart . . . 180

Golf, without cart . . . 240

Gardening, planting flowers . . . 250

Gardening, hoeing & weeding . . . 350

Gardening, digging . . . 500

Ballroom dancing . . . 260

Aerobic dancing . . . 420

Aerobics . . . 450

Step aerobics . . . 550

Skipping rope . . . 700

Walking, 3 mph . . . 280

Jogging, 5mph . . . 500

Hiking . . . 500

Power walking . . . 600

Running . . . 700

Tennis . . . 350

Skating/blading . . . 420

Bicycling, moderate . . . 450

Spinning . . . 650

Squash . . . 650

Water aerobics . . . 400

Swimming . . . 500

Rowing . . . 550

*You can use the Activity Calculator in the online program to determine how many calories you burn while doing dozens more activities.

VEOLIA GIBSON

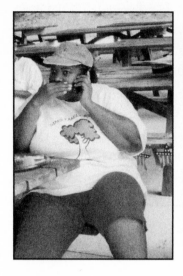 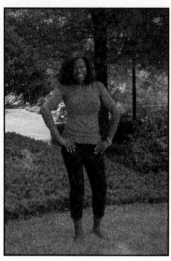

LOST: 252 pounds!

AGE: 54

HEIGHT: 5'8"

BEFORE: 400 pounds, size 32

AFTER: 148 pounds, size 2

◆

THIN ACCOMPLISHMENTS: I love my stamina now, how strong I am. I feel invigorated every day, not exhausted.

THIN CHALLENGES: I finally figured out the right maintenance balance. I eat what I want, but I depend on walking for maintaining or losing. If I go without walking, I'll definitely put weight on.

WORDS OF WISDOM: We need to love ourselves, no matter what. Even at 400 pounds, I was happy with myself. Nothing was dependent on me being a certain size. I just decided I was going to make certain changes to be healthier, and that worked.

WHAT WAS YOUR MOMENT OF REVELATION ABOUT HEALTHY EATING?

I was working as a nanny, and the little boy and I were eating macaroni and cheese. He had two portions and wanted another. The dad said, "You're going to get to eat every day of your life. You don't have to eat all the mac and cheese you want at one sitting." I thought, wow, that's true! I get to eat at least three times a day—I don't have to stuff it all in at once or finish off all the leftovers.

WERE YOU A CLEAN-THE-PLATE KIND OF PERSON?

I didn't just clean the plates. I cleaned everyone else's plates, too. It used to be I didn't like to see food go to waste. I felt it was sinful to throw away food when there were starving children in Africa, so I ate their portions, too! So instead of food going to waste, I added it to my W-A-I-S-T. I still haven't learned to throw food away, but I prepare less, and I store leftovers in the fridge.

DO YOU EXERCISE?

I discovered I love walking, and I'm committed to doing it. It's like leaving home without a shower—I'm not going to do it. How much I walk depends on the "mode" I'm in. Right now, I just got back from my family reunion. I put on a few pounds, so I'm in "reduction mode." That means I walk 8 miles. When I'm in maintenance mode, I only do 2 to 4 miles. If I do more than that, I end up losing more weight than I want.

ON THE IMPORTANCE OF HEALTHY EATING . . .

Ultimately, it's our hearts that matter, but our bodies are a precious gift. If someone gave you a fancy new car and the manual said to use only premium unleaded gas, would you put diesel in it? You have to fuel it—and your body—with the right thing because you want it to run for a really long time.

JOY'S LESSONS LEARNED

NO MEAL IS THE LAST MEAL OF YOUR LIFE. *Another is right around the corner—literally a few hours away. Before you reach for a second helping, or load your plate to overflowing at an all-you-can-eat buffet, or nibble mindlessly from the party appetizer platter, remind yourself that there will be other opportunities to eat. Food will always be there. This moment of desire will pass, but your body will be with you forever!*

Joy's LIFE Diet FAQs

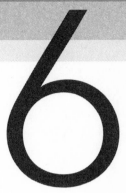

#1: How much weight can I expect to lose?

You can expect to see a dramatic drop on the scale during the first one to three weeks. As for total weight, everyone is a little different. The amount of weight you can expect to lose depends on how much need to lose, how much you were eating before you started the plan, how much exercise you're willing to commit to doing each day, your genetics, your height, your gender, and many other factors.

Since the onset of this program, **LIFE dieters have lost between 3 and 11 pounds during the first week**. How encouraging and invigorating is that! Once your body gets used to the plan, you can expect to lose about 6 to 10 pounds each month until you hit your goal weight.

#2: I work full time plus have kids . . . how can I manage all the kitchen prep involved with this diet plan?

Good question. I'm in the same boat, so I can certainly relate. Please know I created this plan to accommodate ALL types of people and personalities.

If you love variety and have the time to invest, you're in luck. I provide a wide array of recipes and creative ideas for jazzing up your sandwiches and salads. If you don't have a lot of extra time to invest in kitchen prep, you're also in luck. In each step, check out my Easiest Meals At-A-Glance—the simplest (but still delicious!) meals for breakfast, lunch and dinner. For Step One's easy meals see page 55, you'll find Step Two's easy meals on pages 115–116, and Step Three's on pages 200–201.

#3: What if I only like certain foods?

Repeat, repeat, and repeat. You may repeat ANY meal or snack within your appropriate step as often as you'd like. You can literally have the same breakfast everyday. So if you find one or two (or hopefully at least three) that you enjoy, repeat them every morning. If you only like green beans, eat them every single night. You don't have to eat anything you don't like.

I've polled thousands and thousands of people in order to create menus that appeal to every conceivable taste bud, so no matter how picky or limited you are, there will be food you'll enjoy. I've even included a lot of those well-loved home-made classics, such as chicken parmesan and shepherd's pie, as well as everyday standards, such as cereal, oatmeal, turkey sandwiches, and omelets.

#4: This diet seems so expensive

I can understand why it might seem expensive at first glance, but it doesn't have to cost you more than you're spending on groceries now. First, remember that you will be spending less on junk food, so that money goes back into the grocery budget. Beyond that, here are some tips for cutting costs in Joy's LIFE Diet:

- ✦ Make protein swaps—that's what the Approved Foods list is for. If sirloin steak and wild salmon aren't in your budget, swap for lower cost items like skinless chicken, turkey burgers, etc.
- ✦ Buy family packs of chicken, or other items on the Approved Foods list. If you have the room in your freezer, make the initial dollar investment and

get large bags at the wholesale clubs. They may cost you more initially, but less in the long run.

✦ Use frozen veggies and fruits—they are often less expensive than fresh, and just as nutritious. (Just make sure they contain no added anything!)

✦ All non-starchy vegetables are exchangeable, so if a recipe calls for balsamic roasted asparagus and it's January when asparagus is $5.99 a bundle, swap for another veggie, such as carrots. If the meal plan suggests steamed snow peas, but broccoli is on sale that week, by all means save yourself a few bucks and enjoy the broccoli instead.

✦ Use fruit that's in season—Bananas, apples, pears, and oranges are all fine choices in the winter . . . and in summer take advantage of fresh peaches, plums, and berries.

✦ Stock up on canned and packaged staples when they are on sale, especially canned tuna (light in water), canned chicken breast, canned crab, canned salmon (wild or Alaskan, with or without skin and bones, that's your personal choice), oatmeal, and cereal (anything that's on sale will work as long as it fits my criteria: 150 calories or less per 1 cup serving; 8 grams or less sugar; 3+grams fiber)

#5: If my family doesn't have to lose weight, can they eat the same foods?

Definitely! I include recipes for yummy (and healthy) family favorites, such as turkey cheddar burgers, tuna melts, steak, and pita pizzas. If they are not following the plan, you have more freedom to adapt their meals by adding more cheese, different condiments or seasonings, or additional side dishes while still sharing the entrée. These meal options are healthy for everyone, so if your family enjoys them, it's a good thing for the entire gang!

If you cook only for yourself, or if your family is making other choices, I designed recipes with you in mind! Many of my recipes make only a single serving, so they're perfect for just you. But for families—or if you want to cook enough to freeze for later—it is easy enough to double, triple, or quadruple the recipe amounts.

#6: I travel a lot for work, how can I ever stick to this plan?

Joy's LIFE Diet is for all of life, not just the convenient parts. In each step, I give you *LIFE* Restaurant Options, which can help you make diet-friendly choices in any restaurant. In fact, you can lose weight and reach your goal even if you must exclusively dine out. Of course, restaurant ordering is a bit more difficult because you'll be flooded with the sight and aroma of foods to your right and left that are NOT on the plan, but rest assured, you'll know what to order from any menu.

LIFE Restaurant Options for Step One can be found on page 56, for Step Two on pages 116–119, and for Step Three on pages 202–212.

#7: If I'm not hungry in the morning, do I have to eat breakfast?

Most nutrition experts believe that it's important to start your day with a good breakfast, and lots of research bears this out. For instance, a 2005 study showed that when women did not eat breakfast, they took in an average of 100 calories more per day, and had 10% higher levels of insulin, 9% higher total cholesterol, and 17% higher LDL ("bad") cholesterol than when they had a morning meal. At that rate, these women could expect to put on a full ten pounds over the course of a year, *and* to increase their risk of heart disease and diabetes.

Having said that, there *are* people who simply have no appetite in the morning. If your current eating pattern keeps you energized (and doesn't cause overeating at night), then perhaps you really aren't a breakfast person. If that's the case, you may enjoy your LIFE breakfast at any point during the day or skip it completely and double up on your afternoon snack.

#8: Do foods on the Unlimited List, such as celery and cucumbers, really have a negative calorie effect?

By "negative calorie effect," I assume you're asking if the act of chewing certain foods burns up more calories than the food itself contains. Cucumbers and celery top the list of foods rumored to have "negative calorie" value. While it may *seem* like you expend a lot of energy when you chew some things, in reality, chewing eats up only about five measly calories per hour. That being said, all foods on the *LIFE* Unlimited List will certainly help you lose weight . . . not because they create negative calories, but because they're super low-calorie and you're munching on them *instead* of crackers, chips and cookies.

#9: I get intense cravings for chocolate (and potato chips). How can I satisfy these cravings and stay on the LIFE Diet plan?

We all have our moments when we crave special food. For some folks, it's sweet or salty things, and for others it's all about *chocolate*! No matter what your preference, you'll find afternoon snack suggestions that can often do the trick. Also, the following list provides quite a few ideas that can be used towards your daily *LIFE* Extras starting on the first day of Step Two. Items with an asterisk (*) can be eaten starting on the first day of Step Three. For all snacks, be sure to read the labels of packaged items carefully to ensure you're not taking in more than 150 calories.

Sweet Treats

- ✦ One sliced frozen banana
- ✦ One cup grapes, chilled or frozen
- ✦ One cup berries or fruit salad topped with a dollop of reduced-fat whipped topping
- ✦ One low-fat ice cream pop or sandwich
- ✦ One frozen fruit pop
- ✦ 6 ounces plain nonfat yogurt mixed with 2 teaspoons honey
- ✦ Joy Bauer *LIFE* bar
- ✦ *LIFE* muffin
- ✦ *LIFE* smoothie
- ✦ * Lollipop
- ✦ * 100-calorie snack packs (sweet varieties)
- ✦ * Italian ice

Chocolate

- One ounce dark chocolate
- ½ cup low-fat chocolate pudding (any brand, or see LIFE recipe)
- One serving low-fat hot cocoa with any HALF fruit serving
- One low-fat hot cocoa packet mixed with 6 oz nonfat plain or Greek yogurt (semi-frozen or chilled)
- Chocolate covered strawberries: 1 oz dark chocolate melted over 5 whole strawberries
- LIFE Dark Chocolate Cherry muffin
- Joy Bauer LIFE bar
- * Fun size or miniature chocolate bars
- * 100-calorie snack packs (chocolate flavor)
- * 150 calories worth of any chocolate candy

Salty Alternatives

- 150 calories worth of soy crisps or vegetable chips
- 4 cups low-fat popcorn (with or without LIFE seasonings)
- *Half baked potato (white or sweet) topped with salsa and/or nonfat sour cream
- * 150 calories worth of baked potato chips or baked tortilla chips
- * 1-ounce pretzels
- * 100-calorie snack packs (salty cracker/chip varieties)

#10: If I'm hungry after dinner, what should I eat?

You may eat unlimited amounts of food on your Unlimited List at any point during the day or evening. Also, some dinners include HALF a fruit serving, which you may choose to save for later in the evening as well (this allowance is only for dinners which include fruit—you may *not* save other items from breakfast, lunch, or dinner to eat later in the day). Once you hit Step Two, you may also enjoy your

LIFE Extra at any point in the day, so you can choose to save it for after dinner if you like.

#11: I want to gain muscle while I'm reducing fat, so how do I set my target goal?

Unless you're a body builder, muscle doesn't weigh as much as people think in terms of hard pounds.

Here's the math: If you follow a weight training program to build muscle (that's typically 2 to 3 days per week, like the resistance training regimen you're encouraged to follow in Step Three), most people will only average one pound of muscle gain per month . . . and level off when they reach about 3 pounds. So if your weight loss goal is 20 pounds, I say continue to aim for the 20 pound loss . . . and reassess when you hit 17 pounds. Remember, your LIFE goal is to *Look Incredible, Feel Extraordinary*, not fixate on a specific scale number.

#12: Help! I've hit a plateau and my scale has not budged for several weeks.

One of the most common frustrations in weight loss is when all progress seems to screech to a halt and your weight levels off. The one month milestone can be particularly challenging—as the newness of a diet wears off, people tend to loosen up on the reins. In other words, calorie intake tends to sneak back up and we unintentionally scale down on exercise. What's more, your metabolism typically slows down in response to an initial weight loss. Simply put: The smaller you are, the fewer calories you burn.

Here are four simple strategies for breaking through a weight plateau:

1) BOOST YOUR METABOLISM
Since your metabolism naturally slows down as you lose weight, exercise is the obvious way to keep it stoked. If you've been slacking off, get back on track. Even consider adding an extra 10 to 15 minutes of cardio-exercise to your daily

routine—you'll burn at least 50 additional calories. Also, make sure to follow the resistance training exercises (Step Three) two to three days a week. As your weight goes down, you not only lose fat, but also a small amount of muscle. Since muscle is critical to keeping your metabolism revved, losing it can reduce your metabolic rate and hinder weight loss. Strength training in Step Three helps to preserve and build muscle to get your metabolism humming again.

2) CHECK PORTION SIZES AND GET RID OF EXTRAS

After following a diet for a few weeks, we often loosen up and begin to pick and grab. It's amazing how much extra food we can munch on without realizing it, so try to eat mindfully and consider keeping a food log for accountability. Also, pay attention to your beverages (alcohol included), as well as what's going into your coffee and tea. And get out your measuring cups and food scale again. Most dieters routinely underestimate portion sizes.

3) GO BACK ON STEP ONE FOR ONE WEEK

If you need a way to kick-start weight loss, it may be time to go back to the beginning, eliminate *LIFE* Extras, and reenergize your motivation.

4) EVERYDAY WEIGHT LOSS REMINDERS

Nothing new, but this may be the perfect time to remind you:

Eat slower. Research shows that people eat approximately 60 fewer calories per meal when they slow down the pace. If you count all three meals, that's a big 180 calories every day.

Get at least 7 hours of sleep each night. Sleep deprivation causes an imbalance in certain hormones, which leaves us feeling hungrier during the day, and more likely to ignore a diet.

Plan ahead. Take a few minutes the night before (or when you first get up in the morning) to plan out your food for the day. When you're mentally prepared with a food strategy, you'll be less likely to jump ship.

#13: I have too much belly fat, which my doctor told me is dangerous. Does Joy's LIFE Diet specifically target belly fat first?

Contrary to what some diet books and articles preach, certain foods and diet programs *cannot* magically melt away the fat off your belly (or any other part of your body). Where fat tends to settle is typically all in your genetics.

The good news is when you eat an appropriate amount of calories for weight loss (meaning less than you burn), you'll eventually lose weight "all over" your body—including your personal problem areas, such as your belly, if that's where you have it. And if you add regular exercise to a healthy diet, you'll burn even more calories, and tone, tighten, and strengthen the muscles underneath the fat. That way, when the fat comes off, you'll look even leaner.

#14: People always seem to be pushing food on me—at the office, family gatherings, and parties. What can I do to combat this food peer pressure?

"Food peer pressure" is something we don't often think about, but we have been experiencing it since childhood. In fact, grandmothers and mothers can be some of the most relentless "food pushers." Fortunately, there are ways to stick to my LIFE Diet without making waves at the table. Consider the following:

◆ *Brag about your new-found health effort.* There's a good chance that others will follow your lead—and they'll be less likely to push unhealthy food on you.

◆ *Remember your manners.* Pay attention to the ways in which you phrase things. "No thank you, but that sure looks delicious," or "Thanks so much for offering, but I'm not really hungry right now," are polite ways of passing up a dish. You can even try, "That looks so great. May I have some for later?" These statements will enable you to deny the dish without hurting anyone's feelings.

◆ *Have a taste.* It's OK to try a bite or two. This will also give you the opportunity to praise the cook's work. Just make sure you don't turn this tasting opportunity into a feast.

#15: I heard that if you eat late at night, the food turns straight to fat. But that's when I get hungry. Is it okay if I save my snack for just before bed?

Yes, that's fine. The "food straight to fat" thing is a myth. It's practically guaranteed that if your collective calories—calories eaten throughout the entire day—are appropriate for your personal weight maintenance, you won't gain weight from late night dinners and/or snacks.

On the other hand, if you skip breakfast to "save calories," sacrifice lunch to meetings and phone calls, and then eat a whole day's worth of food for dinner, you have a good chance of gaining weight. Think about it—the body needs energy for its vital functions at all times of day, and energy demands are the greatest when you're most mentally and physically active, which is generally *during* the day. If you chronically run on empty when your body and mind most need fuel, you're bound to stall your metabolism (a set up for weight gain). Besides, the longer you wait to eat, the hungrier you become, and the more likely you are to overeat at night—clearly causing weight gain.

#16: I'm over age 50, and I think my metabolism is shot. Can I still lose weight on Joy's LIFE Diet?

Yes, your metabolism has probably slowed—it naturally slows down for everyone by about 2 to 5% per decade after age 40. But that doesn't mean you're a lost cause! Plenty of women and men have had great success losing weight on my program, regardless of their age. I strongly urge you NOT to skip the exercise portion of the program—exercise can boost your metabolism so that you don't feel so "shot."

#17: I want to try this diet, but I'm never good at these things because I'm an emotional eater. I start strong, but give up too soon. Am I going to have better luck this time?

Emotional eating is very common, and I hear concerns like yours in my practice all the time. People eat in response to any number of uncomfortable feelings, including stress, anxiety, sadness, boredom, anger, loneliness, relationship problems, and poor self-esteem. When emotions (rather than your stomach) determine your eating habits, it can quickly lead to overeating, weight gain, guilt, and—yes—giving up on diets. If you are serious about working on your weight, it is possible to overcome unnecessary eating.

- *Keep a Food/Mood Journal.* Write down your food choices and portions, where you eat, why you eat, how you feel, and anything else that allows you to see your healthy (and unhealthy) patterns. That way, you can identify tough timeframes, spot areas for improvement, and make adjustments as you go along. Use the journal to track your progress as you weigh yourself once or twice a week.
- *Get a Diet Buddy.* Some people do better if they have a friend, spouse, online community, therapist, *someone* they can talk to about successes or setbacks. Ideally, this person is nonjudgmental and unconditionally supportive. If you thrive with a little help from your friends, go ahead and ask for their help and guidance.
- *Start a New Hobby.* Spend less time obsessing over food by redirecting your focus and energy. Pick up quilting, sewing, play tennis, learn a new language, volunteer for a charity—anything goes.
- *Have an Emergency Plan.* Prepare a list of activities that are personally appealing and handy for those times when you are tempted to overeat. Perhaps go for a walk, call a friend, listen to nostalgic music, take a hot shower/bath, clean your house, polish your nails, surf the Internet, schedule outstanding appointments, watch something on TiVo, clean your purse, organize your closet, look through a photo album, etc.

Appendix—
Life Steps in a Nutshell

Meats, Poultry, and Pork

Eat only when designated at a particular meal—and carefully check portions.

STEP ONE	Meats (lean cuts only) Bottom round Buffalo Filet mignon Flank London broil Sirloin Top round Veal Venison Poultry (skinless only) Chicken breast Chicken breast, ground (at least 90% lean) Chicken thigh Cornish hen Ostrich Turkey breast Turkey burger (lean) Turkey thigh Turkey, ground (at least 90% lean) Pork Pork tenderloin
STEP TWO	*all meats, poultry, and pork on Step One, plus:* Poultry Poultry sausage (lean) Turkey bacon Pork Ham, lean
STEP THREE	*all meats, poultry, and pork on Steps One and Two, plus:* Meats Ground sirloin (at least 90% lean) Lean deli roast beef Pork Canadian bacon

Fish and Seafood

Eat only when designated at a particular meal—and carefully check portions.

STEP ONE	Anchovies Catfish Clams Cod Crab (fresh or canned) Flounder Haddock Halibut Lobster Mackerel (Atlantic only, not king) Mahi mahi Mussels Oysters Red snapper Salmon, wild (fresh and canned) Sardines Scallops Shrimp Sole Tilapia Trout Tuna (canned light in water) Whitefish
STEP TWO	*all fish and seafood on Step One, plus:* Imitation crab meat Lox Smoked salmon
STEP THREE	*all fish and seafood on Steps One and Two*

Eggs, Vegan Proteins, and Dairy

Eat only when designated at a particular meal—and carefully check portions.

STEP ONE	**Eggs**
	   Egg whites
	   Egg substitute
	Vegan Proteins
	   Soy milk (low-fat)
	   Soy yogurt (nonfat and low-fat)
	   Tempeh
	   Tofu
	   Vegan cheese (nonfat and low-fat)
	   Veggie burgers
	   Wheat gluten/seitan
	Dairy
	   Cheese, fat-free (all varieties)
	   Cheese, reduced-fat (all varieties)
	   Cheese, Parmesan
	   Cheese, Romano
	   Greek yogurt (nonfat)
	   Yogurt, nonfat plain and vanilla (no artificial sweetener)

STEP TWO	*all eggs, vegan proteins, and dairy on Step One, plus:*
	Eggs
	   Eggs, whole
	Dairy
	   Yogurt, nonfat plain and flavored (all brands 100 calories or less)

STEP THREE	*all eggs, vegan proteins, and dairy on Steps One and Two, plus:*
	Dairy
	   Cheese, Feta
	   Cheese, Gorgonzola

Vegetables

While you can have unlimited portions of non-starchy vegetables, be sure to eat starchy vegetables only when designated at a particular meal—and carefully check portions.

	Non-starchy vegetables (unlimited amounts)
	Artichokes and artichoke hearts
	Asparagus
	Beans, non-starchy: green, yellow, Italian, and wax
	Beets
	Bok choy (Chinese cabbage)
	Broccoli
	Broccoli rabe
	Broccolini
	Brussels sprouts
	Cabbage
	Carrots
	Cauliflower
	Celery
	Dark green leafy vegetables:
	Beet greens
	Collard greens
STEP ONE	Dandelion greens
	Kale
	Mustard greens
	Spinach
	Swiss chard
	Turnip greens
	Eggplant
	Fennel
	Garlic
	Green onions (scallions)
	Jicama
	Leeks
	Lettuce:
	Arugula
	Endive
	Escarole
	Iceberg
	Mixed greens/salad blends
	Romaine
	(continued)

	Mixed vegetable blends without corn, starchy beans, peas, pasta, or any kind of sauce
	Mushrooms
	Okra
	Onions
	Peppers (all varieties)
	Pickles
	Pumpkin (fresh, frozen, or canned—must say "100% pure pumpkin," no sugar added)
	Radicchio
	Radishes
	Red peppers, roasted (if packed in oil, pat dry)
	Rhubarb
	Sea vegetables (nori, etc.)
	Shallots
	Snow peas
	Spaghetti squash
	Sprouts (all varieties)
	Summer (yellow) squash
	Tomato
	Water chestnuts
	Watercress
	Zucchini
STEP TWO	*all vegetables on Step One, plus: **Non-starchy vegetables** Sauerkraut **Starchy vegetables (NOT unlimited—carefully check portions)** Beans (legumes) Green peas Lentils Sweet potato
STEP THREE	*all vegetables on Steps One and Two, plus: **Starchy vegetables (NOT unlimited—carefully check portions)** Corn White potato

Whole Grains

Eat only when designated at a particular meal—and carefully check portions.

STEP ONE	Mini whole grain pita bread (no more than 70 calories) Reduced calorie whole grain bread (no more than 45 calories per slice) Rice cakes (stick with plain, 45 calories per rick cake) Wheat germ Whole grain bread (any brand that lists "whole wheat" as first ingredient) Whole grain cereal (any brand 150 calories or less per 1 cup serving; no more than 8 grams sugar; at least 3 grams fiber) Whole grain oats (plain flavor only; traditional, quick cooking, or steel-cut oats)
STEP TWO	*all whole grains on Step One, plus:* Whole grain English muffin (any brand 130 calories or less) *LIFE* Muffins Whole grain tortilla wrap (no more than 100 calories per wrap) Regular whole grain pita bread (150 calories or less) Whole grain waffles (no more than 170 calories per two waffles)
STEP THREE	*all whole grains on Steps One and Two, plus:* Joy Bauer *LIFE* Bars Whole grain pasta Brown rice Whole grain couscous Hotdog buns (preferably whole grain) Bread crumbs (preferably whole grain) Taco shells (soft or hard)

Fruit: HALF and WHOLE Fruit Serving Options

Eat fruit only when designated for a particular meal, and be careful to pick from the right serving size when making substitutions.

		HALF Serving	WHOLE Serving
STEP ONE	Apple	1 small (palm-sized)	1 large
	Apricot, dried	6 halves	12 halves
	Apricot, fresh	3 large	6 large
	Banana	½	1
	Berries (fresh or frozen, unsweetened blueberries, raspberries, blackberries, boysenberries, or sliced medium-sized strawberries)	¾ cup or 10 whole medium-sized strawberries	1½ cups or 20 whole medium-sized strawberries
	Cantaloupe	¼ medium or 1 cup cubed	½ medium or 2 cups cubed
	Cherries, fresh	½ cup or 10 whole	1 cup or 20 whole
	Clementines	1	2
	Fruit salad, fresh cut (from the produce section, unsweetened)	½ cup	1 cup
	Grapefruit (red, pink, or white)	½	1 whole
	Grapes, seedless (red, purple, green, or black)	½ cup	1 cup
	Honeydew melon, cubed	1 cup	2 cups

		HALF Serving	WHOLE Serving
	Kiwi, large	1	2
	Mango	½ fresh or ½ cup chunks (unsweetened)	1 medium fresh or 1 cup chunks (unsweetened)
	Nectarine	1	2
	Orange, medium	1	2
	Papaya, fresh cubed	1 cup	2 cups
	Peach, large	1	2
	Pear	½ large or 1 small	1 large
	Pineapple chunks, fresh	½ cup	1 cup
	Plum	2 small or 1 large	2 large
	Pomegranate	½ medium	1 medium
	Prunes, large	3	6
	Raisins	2 tablespoons	¼ cup
	Tangerine, medium	1	2
	Watermelon, cubed	1 cup	2 cups
STEP TWO	*all fruits on Step One		
STEP THREE	*all fruits on Step One		

Seasonings, Condiments, Marinades, and Healthy Fats

Use these items to jazz up your meals. For all items that do NOT appear on the Unlimited list (salad dressings, ketchup, mayonnaise, olive oil, nut butters, avocado, etc.), eat only when designated at a meal or snack and be sure to stick with the specific portion listed.

STEP ONE	Avocado Chiles or hot peppers, fresh or canned in vinegar/water Extracts (vanilla, almond, peppermint, etc.) Horseradish Hot sauce Ketchup Lemon, fresh Lime, fresh Marinara sauce (opt for brands with 60 calories or less per half cup serving) Mayonnaise, reduced-fat (any brand, 25 calories or less per tablespoon) Mustard (plain, brown, spicy, Dijon) Nonstick cooking spray (any variety) Nuts (almonds and pistachios) Nut butters (peanut, soy, almond, etc.) Olive oil Salad dressing, Caesar (only use for Caesar salad lunch option—any brand, no more than 80 calories per 2 tablespoons) Salad dressing, low-calorie (any brand with no more than 40 calories per 2 tablespoons) Salad dressing, any of Joy's LIFE recipes Salsa (mild or spicy; any brand without added sugar or corn syrup) Salt substitute Soy sauce, low-sodium Teriyaki sauce, low-sodium Vinegar, any type—not vinaigrette Wasabi Herbs and spices

	Allspice, anise seed, basil, bay leaves, cardamom, cayenne pepper, celery seed, chili powder, Chinese five-spice, chives, cilantro, cinnamon, cloves, coriander, cumin, curry powder, dill weed, garlic powder, ginger, lemongrass, marjoram, mint, mustard, mustard seed, nutmeg, Old Bay seasoning, onion powder, oregano, paprika, parsley, pepper (ground) and whole peppercorns, pumpkin pie spice, red pepper flakes, rosemary, sage, seasoning blends (without added sugar or salt), tarragon, thyme, and turmeric
STEP TWO	*all seasonings, condiments, marinades, and healthy fats on Step One, plus:* Fruit jam Honey Maple syrup (real or reduced sugar/calorie) Olives Orange juice, 100% juice Steak sauce Sugar, brown or white Worcestershire sauce
STEP THREE	*all seasonings, condiments, marinades, and healthy fats on Steps One and Two, plus:* Barbecue sauce (any brand, 40 calories or less per 2 tablespoons) Capers Chili sauce Sesame seeds Tomato juice

Beverages

Enjoy any time of day.

STEP ONE	Club soda Coffee (no artificial sweeteners or natural sweeteners, including sugar. No cream or whole milk. You may add skim, 1%, or low-fat/light soy milk only) Naturally flavored zero-calorie coffee with no natural or artificial sweeteners Seltzer, zero calorie (plain and naturally flavored) Sparkling water Tea—black, white, green, herbal (no artificial sweeteners or natural sweeteners, including sugar or honey) Water Naturally flavored waters, calorie-free
STEP TWO	*all beverages on Step One, plus:* Diet soda and other artificially sweetened beverages (each 12-ounce can or 20-ounce bottle counts as half of your daily artificial sweetener allotment)
STEP THREE	*all beverages on Steps One and Two*

Acceptable Mid-Afternoon Snack List

You may substitute afternoon snacks listed on your menu with the following options within each step. Stick with one per day, and keep an eye on designated portions.

STEP ONE	**Cheese Options** ✦ 1 ounce reduced-fat or fat-free cheese with unlimited celery and pepper sticks ✦ 1 ounce reduced-fat or fat-free cheese with 1 mini whole-grain pita or rice cake ✦ 1 ounce reduced-fat or fat-free cheese with 10 raw almonds or 15 pistachio nuts ✦ 1 part-skim cheese stick with a HALF fruit serving ✦ 4 level tablespoons reduced-fat cream cheese with unlimited celery sticks ✦ ½ cup low-fat or nonfat cottage cheese, topped with a HALF fruit serving ✦ ½ cup low-fat or nonfat cottage cheese with unlimited non-starchy vegetables (i.e., cherry tomatoes, red pepper strips, celery, or baby carrots) ✦ ¾ cup low-fat or nonfat cottage cheese, plain or with cinnamon ✦ 1 slice reduced calorie, whole-grain toast with 1 ounce slice reduced or nonfat cheese and optional tomato slices ✦ 1 slice reduced calorie, whole-grain toast (any brand 45 calories or less per slice) with 1 level tablespoon reduced-fat cream cheese **Yogurt Options** ✦ 8 ounces nonfat plain, Greek, or vanilla yogurt (no artificial sweeteners) ✦ 6 ounces nonfat plain or Greek yogurt (no artificial sweeteners), topped with 2 tablespoons wheat germ or ground flaxseed ✦ 6 ounces nonfat plain or Greek yogurt (no artificial sweeteners), topped with a HALF fruit serving **Nut and Nut Butter Options** ✦ 10 raw almonds or 15 pistachios and a HALF fruit serving ✦ 10 raw almonds or 15 pistachios and ½ cup (one snack container) no-sugar-added natural applesauce ✦ 20 raw almonds ✦ 30 pistachios ✦ 2 level teaspoons natural peanut butter and a HALF fruit serving, i.e., ½ banana or 1 small apple

	✦ 1 level tablespoon natural peanut butter with unlimited celery sticks ✦ 1 slice reduced calorie, whole-grain toast (any brand 45 calories or less per slice) with 1 level tablespoon natural peanut butter **Fruit Options** ✦ 1 frozen banana ✦ 1 cup frozen grapes ✦ One WHOLE fruit serving ✦ 1 orange (or any other HALF fruit serving) and 1 mini whole-grain pita **Miscellaneous Options** ✦ 4 ounces turkey breast rolled with lettuce and mustard ✦ 1 mini whole-grain pita with 2 level tablespoons hummus (any variety) ✦ ¼ cup hummus (any variety) with unlimited cucumber slices, celery sticks, and/or red, yellow, and green bell pepper strips ✦ 1 cup edamame beans boiled in the pod (green soybeans, fresh or frozen)
STEP TWO	*all mid-afternoon snacks on Step One, plus:* **Yogurt Options** ✦ 8 ounces flavored yogurt (any brand 150 calories or less) ✦ 6 ounces flavored yogurt (any brand 100 calories or less), topped with 2 tablespoons wheat germ or ground flaxseed ✦ 6 ounces flavored yogurt (any brand 100 calories or less), topped with a HALF fruit serving ✦ Vanilla Pumpkin Pudding: 6 ounces nonfat vanilla yogurt (any brand 100 calories or less) mixed with ½ cup 100% pure pumpkin puree and cinnamon to taste **Fruit Options** ✦ 1 *LIFE* Smoothie **Miscellaneous Options** ✦ ½ medium ripe avocado drizzled with lime juice, salt and pepper to taste ✦ 1 rice cake+one hard boiled egg (or 4 egg whites) ✦ 1 slice reduced calorie whole-grain toast (any brand 45 calories or less per slice) topped with one hard boiled egg mashed and mixed with minced onion and 1 teaspoon reduced-fat mayonnaise. ✦ 1 *LIFE* Muffin ✦ 1 Joy Bauer *LIFE Bar*

STEP THREE

all mid-afternoon snacks on Steps One and Two, plus:

Cheese Options

+ ½ cup low-fat or nonfat cottage cheese mixed with ½ cup canned crushed pineapple (canned in its own juice and drained)
+ 1 dry toasted whole-grain English muffin (any brand 130 calories or less) topped with 2 teaspoons fat-free cream cheese

Yogurt Options

+ Bananas and Cream: 6 ounces nonfat vanilla yogurt (any brand 100 calories or less) mixed with ½ banana, thinly sliced

Nuts and Nut Butter Options

+ 2 rice cakes (any brand 45 calories or less per cake)+one teaspoon peanut, almond, apple, or soy nut butter

Fruit Options

+ Banana Split: 1 banana, split lengthwise and topped with 2 tablespoons reduced-fat whipped topping
+ 12-ounce skim latte or cappuccino with optional 1 teaspoon/packet sugar or artificial sweetener+small apple (or any HALF fruit serving)

Vegetable Options

+ Half a small-medium baked potato (sweet or white) topped with 2 tablespoons salsa, ketchup, or nonfat sour cream
+ 1 regular whole wheat pita (or 2 mini pitas), cut into wedges, sprayed with nonstick cooking spray, and baked at 375°F for 10 to 15 minutes+2 tablespoons salsa
+ Curry Sweet Potato Fries
+ 2 cups *LIFE* soup with 1 mini whole wheat pita (any brand 70 calories or less per pita) *or* 1 slice reduced calorie whole wheat toast (any brand 45 calories or less per slice) *or* 60–70 calories worth of whole grain crackers
+ Spinach or Broccoli Marinara: Microwave one 10-ounce package frozen chopped spinach or broccoli until cooked. Thoroughly drain and mix with 2 heaping tablespoons marinara sauce. Place back in microwave and reheat for 45 seconds. Top with optional 2 tablespoons parmesan or reduced-fat shredded cheese.

Miscellaneous Options

+ Hummus "Deviled" Eggs: 2 hard boiled eggs, halved lengthwise and yolks replaced with a total of ¼ cup hummus (any variety)
+ 150 calories worth of soy crisps (any flavor variety)
+ 4 cups low-fat popcorn (any prepared or microwaveable brand 30 calories or less per cup, with or without low-calorie *LIFE* seasoning blends).

Unlimited Food/Beverage List

Enjoy in unlimited amounts—at any time of the day.

STEP ONE	ALL non-starchy vegetables! Club soda (with optional fresh lemon or lime) Coffee (black, or with skim, 1%, or low-fat/light soy milk only; no natural or artificial sweeteners) Naturally flavored zero-calorie coffee with no natural or artificial sweeteners Extracts (vanilla, almond, peppermint, etc.) Herbs and spices Horseradish Hot sauce Lemon and lime wedges Low-sodium broth Mustard (plain, brown, spicy, Dijon) Nonstick cooking spray Joy's *LIFE* Balsamic Vinaigrette Salad Dressing Salt substitute Seltzer, zero calorie (plain and naturally flavored) Sparkling water Tea (iced or hot, with lemon or skim, 1%, or low-fat/light soy milk only; no natural or artificial sweeteners) Vinegar (any variety) Wasabi Water (with optional fresh lemon or lime) Naturally flavored waters, zero-calorie
STEP TWO	*all unlimited food/beverages on Step One, plus:* Salsa (mild or spicy; any brand without added sugar or corn syrup) Sauerkraut Soy sauce, low-sodium Worcestershire sauce
STEP THREE	*all unlimited food/beverages on Steps One and Two, plus:* Sugar-free gum

afternoon snack, 283–84
   Step One, 21, 38–40, 303–304
   Step Three, 153, 170–73, 179–99, 305
   Step Two, 78, 94–96, 101–114, 304
alcohol, 20, 22, 75
Almonds, Savory, 133
Alternating Back Lunges, 269–70
apple:
   Apple Cinnamon Pancakes with Yogurt Topping, 124–25
   Chicken-Apple Salad Chop, 128
   LIFE Apple Cinnamon Muffins, 119
artificial sweeteners, 20, 23, 74

Balsamic Vinaigrette, 60
banana:
   LIFE Banana Blueberry Muffins, 123
   LIFE Banana Cardamom Smoothie, 132
   LIFE Strawberry Banana Smoothie, 132
barley, 22

beans, 5, 22
   Uncle Onion's Turkey Bean Chile, 222
Beef Teriyaki, 65–66
beer, 22
belly fat, 287
berries, 34
   frozen vs. fresh, 34
beverages, 286
   Step One, 37–38, 41, 302, 306
   Step Three, 170, 174, 302, 306
   Step Two, 94, 96–97, 132–37, 302, 306
binge, 238
Bird Dog, 262
bloating, 3, 16, 254
blood flow, 244
blood pressure, 19, 244
blueberry:
   Blueberry Mango Sorbet, 135
   LIFE Banana Blueberry Muffins, 123
   LIFE Blueberry Mango Smoothie, 132
Boston Market, 210
brain chemistry, 245
bread, 5, 22

breakfast, 7–8
  importance of, 282
  protein substitutions, 86, 161
  recipes, 57–58, 119–26, 213–14
  skipping, 282, 288
  Step One, 21, 26–34, 48–56, 57–58
  Step Three, 153, 158–67, 179–99, 202, 213–14
  Step Two, 78, 82–91, 101–115, 117
Breakfast Pizza, 125
Broccoli & Cheese Omelet, 59
buckwheat, 22
buddy system, 9, 13, 72, 250, 289
Burger, E-Z Turkey, 68
Burger King, 204–205
Burger with Sautéed Mushrooms, Cheddar Turkey, 68
Burrito Pocket, Skinny, 58

Caesar Dressing, 61
calcium, 18–19
calorie burn, 244
cancer, 244, 245
canned foods, 281
carbohydrates, 5
Cardamom Smoothie, LIFE Banana, 132
cardiovascular exercise, 254–60
Carlson, Patti, 175–76
Carrot Spice Muffins, LIFE, 121
Cauliflower Mashed "Potatoes," 69
cells, 5
cereals, 5, 22, 25
changing your life, 1–9
Cheddar Turkey Burger with Sautéed Mushrooms, 68
cheese:
  afternoon snacks, 38–39, 94–95, 171, 303, 305
  Broccoli & Cheese Omelet, 59
  Easy Cheesy Salmon Melt, 216
  Egg-Cellent Omelet with Vegetables & Cheese, 57

  Ham and Cheese Omelet with Chives, 126
  See also specific cheeses
Cherry Muffins, LIFE Dark Chocolate, 122
Chesapeake Shrimp Boil, 138
chicken, 280
  Chicken-Apple Salad Chop, 128
  Chicken Florentine, 140
  Chicken Salad, 217
  Chicken Sloppy Joes, 225
  Chicken Teriyaki, 67
  Curried Chicken Salad with Sweet Green Peas, 127
  Easy Chicken Puttanesca, 139
  Gorgonzola-Walnut Stuffed Chicken Breast, 225–26
  Grilled Chicken Parmesan, 69
  Sweet and Sour Chicken, 228
  See also poultry
Chick-fil-A, 211–12
chickpeas, 22
Chili, Uncle Onion's Turkey Bean, 222
Chipotle, 212–13
chocolate, 75, 76, 284
  cravings, 283, 284
  Creamy Chocolate Pudding, 136
  LIFE Dark Chocolate Cherry Muffins, 122
cholesterol, 19, 244, 282
Cinnamon Muffins, LIFE Apple, 119
Cinnamon Pancakes with Yogurt Topping, Apple, 124–25
Circuit Workout, 267–72
  Alternating Back Lunges, 269–70
  Modified Push-Ups, 270
  Seated Reverse Fly, 271–72
  Seated Rows, 271
  Side-to-Side Lunges, 269–70
  Sumo Squats, 269
Cobra Stretch, 265
cocoa, 75, 76
Cod, Crispy Oven Fried, 219–20

coffee, 41
    Funky Monkey Coffee Drink, 137
    naturally flavored zero-calorie, 37
Coleslaw for One, Creamy, 218
commitment, 13
compulsions, 81
condiments, 34
    Step One, 34–36, 300–301
    Step Three, 167–70, 301
    Step Two, 91–93, 301
Cook, Devyn, 24–25
corn, 22
cost of food, 280–81
Crab Salad, 215
cravings, food, 283–84
Creamsicle Smoothie, LIFE, 133
Creamy Chocolate Pudding, 136
Creamy Coleslaw for One, 218
Creamy Garlic Dill Dressing, 63
Creamy Vanilla Pudding, 136
Crispy Oven Fried Cod, 219–20
Curried Chicken Salad with Sweet Green
    Peas, 127
Curry Sweet Potato Fried, 220

dairy products, 5
    portion sizes, 45
    Step One, 29, 294
    Step Three, 162, 294
    Step Two, 85, 294
    See also specific dairy products
Dead Bugs, 263
diabetes, 19, 244
diet soft drinks, 20, 23
Dijon Dressing, Maple, 63
Dijon Pork Tenderloin, Orange, 144
Dill Dressing, Creamy Garlic, 63
Dill Sauce, Microwave Poached Salmon
    with Lemon, 219
dinner, 284–85, 288
    no starch with, 20, 22
    recipes, 59–69, 137–44, 218–28

Step One, 21, 26–34, 48–56, 59–69
Step Three, 153, 158–67, 179–99,
    203–204
Step Two, 78, 82–91, 101–115, 118–19,
    137–44
Dinowitz, Howard, 7981
disease, 19, 244, 245, 250
Domino's Pizza, 210–11
Doorway Stretch, 264
Dreher, Lisa, 43–44
dressings, 34, 60–63
    Balsamic Vinaigrette, 60
    Caesar, 61
    Creamy Garlic Dill, 63
    Maple Dijon, 63
    Orange Ginger, 62
    Raspberry Vinaigrette, 61
    Thousand Island, 61
    Tomato Parmesan, 62

Easiest Meals At-A-Glance, 280
    Step One, 55
    Step Three, 200–201
    Step Two, 115–16
Easy Cheesy Salmon Melt, 216
Easy Chicken Puttanesca, 139
eating style, changing, 3–4
Egg-cellent Omelet with Vegetables &
    Cheese, 57
eggs:
    Egg White Salad, 215
    Fiesta Scrambled Eggs with Green
        Chiles, 213
    LIFE Quiche, 137–38
    Loaded Veggie Frittata, 226
    Spinach and Feta Egg Scramble,
        214
    Step One, 29, 294
    Step Three, 161, 294
    Step Two, 84, 294
    See also omelet
emotional eating, 253, 288–89

energy, 3, 16

enzymes, 7

exercise, 21, 243–77, 285–86, 287, 288

   benefits of, 243–46

   calorie burning chart by activity, 274

   cardiovascular, 254–60

   Circuit Workout, 267–72

   LIFE Enhancers, 261–65, 268, 269

   low-impact, 255

   resistance training, 267–72, 285

   Step Four, 273–74

   Step One, 254–60

   Step Three, 266–72

   Step Two, 260–66

   thinking positively about, 249–51

   walking, 254–60, 261

   See also specific exercises

expectations:

   LIFE, 2–4

   weight loss, 279

E-Z Turkey Burger, 68

family, cooking for, 281

FAQs, LIFE Diet, 279–89

fast food, Step Three options, 204–213

fats, 5, 34

   portion sizes, 46

   Step One, 34–36, 300–301

   Step Three, 167–70, 301

   Step Two, 91–93, 301

fava beans, 22

feta:

   Greek Salad with, 217

   Spinach and Feta Egg Scramble, 214

fiber, 5

Fiesta Scrambled Eggs with Green Chiles, 213

fight-or-flight response, 249, 250

fish and seafood, 5, 6

   cost of, 280, 281

Fish Fillet en Papillote with Garden Vegetables, 223

   Step One, 28–29, 293

   Step Three, 160, 293

   Step Two, 84, 293

   See also specific fish and seafood

fish oil, 19

French Toast, Vanilla, 213–14

Fries, Curry Sweet Potato, 220

frozen meals, 74

fruits, 5, 75

   afternoon snack, 40, 95–96, 172, 304, 305

   cost of, 281

   frozen vs. fresh, 34

   off season, 34

   Step One, 32–34, 40, 298–99

   Step Three, 165–67, 172, 299

   Step Two, 89–91, 95–96, 299

   See also specific fruits

Funky Monkey Coffee Drink, 137

Garlic Dill Dressing, Creamy, 63

Garlic Shrimp, Lemon, 224

Gibson, Veolia, 275–76

ginger:

   Ginger Lime Salmon Cakes, 224–25

   LIFE Mango Ginger Muffins, 120

   Orange Ginger Dressing, 62

goals, 236

Gorgonzola-Walnut Stuffed Chicken Breast, 225–26

Granita, Grapefruit Rosemary, 135

Grapefruit Rosemary Granita, 135

Greek Salad with Feta, 217

Green Chiles, Fiesta Scrambled Eggs with, 213

Green Peas, Curried Chicken Salad with Sweet, 127

Grilled Chicken Parmesan, 69

Grosse, Pam & David, 70–72

gum, sugarless, 40

habits, bad, 3–4
Halbrook, Annette, 145–46
Halibut Kebabs, Tandoori, 141
Ham and Cheese Omelet with Chives, 126
Haraldson-Bering, Lynn, 240–41
Hardee's, 211
heart disease, 19, 244, 250
heart rate, 256
    monitor, 257
hobbies, 289
hormones, 7, 16

ice cream, 25
inflammation, 5
iron, 18

Jamba Juice, 210
journal, food, 9, 289

Kebabs, Halibut, 141
ketchup, 34
KFC, 211
kitchen prep, 279–80
Klementsen, Tory & Roy, 10, *10*, 11–13

labels, food, 152
Lemon Dill Sauce, Microwave Poached
    Salmon with, 219
Lemon Garlic Shrimp, 224
lentils, 22
Letts, Melissa, 155–57
LIFE Apple Cinnamon Muffins, 119
LIFE Banana Blueberry Muffins, 123
LIFE Banana Cardamom Smoothie, 132
LIFE Blueberry Mango Smoothie, 132
LIFE Carrot Spice Muffins, 121
LIFE Creamsicle Smoothie, 133
LIFE Dark Chocolate Cherry Muffins,
    122

LIFE Diet:
    exercise and, 243–77
    expectations, 2–4
    FAQs, 279–89
    four steps, 6
    Step Four (Reveal), 6, 231–42
    Step One (Release), 6, 15–72
    Step Three (Relearn), 6, 149–230
    Step Two (Relearn), 6, 73–147
LIFE Dinner Salad, 59–60
LIFE Enhancers, 260, 261–65, 268, 269
    Bird Dog, 262
    Cobra Stretch, 265
    Dead Bugs, 263
    Doorway Stretch, 264
    Neck Stretches, 265
    Pelvic Bridges, 263
    Walking Into Walls, 264
LIFE Healthy Extras, 74, 75–76, 151, 152,
    178, 237–38, 283
LIFE Mango Ginger Muffins, 120
LIFE Oatmeal Pancake, 126
LIFE Quiche, 137–38
LIFE Scallion Pancake with Sour Cream,
    218
LIFE Shepherd's Pie, 143
LIFE Strawberry Banana Smoothie,
    132–33
LIFE Veggie Soup, 63–65
Lime, Shrimp Ceviche with, 142
Lime Salmon Cakes, Ginger, 224–25
Loaded Veggie Frittata, 226
low-impact exercise, 255
loyalties, food, 4
lunch, 288
    recipes, 58–59, 127–31, 137–44,
        215–18
    Step One, 21, 26–34, 48–56, 58–59
    Step Three, 153, 158–67, 179–99,
        202–203, 215–18
    Step Two, 78, 82–91, 101–115, 117–18,
        127–31
Lusk, Sissy, 247–48

mango:
  Blueberry Mango Sorbet, 135
  LIFE Blueberry Mango Smoothie, 132
  LIFE Mango Ginger Muffins, 120
Maple Dijon Dressing, 63
marinades, 34
  Step One, 34–36, 300–301
  Step Three, 167–70, 301
  Step Two, 91–93, 301
mayo, 34
McDonald's, 205–206
meat, 6
  cost of, 280–81
  Step One, 27, 292
  Step Three, 159, 292
  Step Two, 83, 292
  See also specific meats
Meatloaves, Mini Turkey, 221
memory, 3, 245
men, 47, 100, 177
menus and recipes:
  Step One, 47–69
  Step Three, 177–228
  Step Two, 100–144
  See also specific recipes
metabolism, 288
  boosting, 285–86
Microwave Poached Salmon with Lemon
  Dill Sauce, 219
Mielarczyk, Janice, 98–99
mind, changing your, 3
Minestrone Soup, 131
Mini Turkey Meatloaves, 221
Mint Tea, Summer, 41
Modified Push-Ups, 270
monounsaturated fats, 5
mood, 16, 289
  emotional eating, 253, 288–89
  swings, 3
Morrison, Marilyn, 145–46
motivation, 8–9
muffins:
  LIFE Apple Cinnamon, 119

LIFE Banana Blueberry, 123
LIFE Carrot Spice, 121
LIFE Dark Chocolate Cherry, 122
LIFE Mango Ginger, 120
muscles, 244, 267, 285, 286
mushrooms:
  Cheddar Turkey Burger with Sautéed
    Mushrooms, 68
  Stuffed Portobello Mushroom Caps, 227
music, 9
mustard, 34
  Maple Dijon Dressing, 63
  Orange Dijon Pork Tenderloin, 144

Neck Stretches, 265
"negative" calories, 282–83
nighttime snack, 7, 8, 44, 284–85, 288
nut butter, 39, 95, 172, 303, 304, 305
nuts, 5, 75
  afternoon snack, 39, 95, 172, 303–305
  See also specific nuts

Oatmeal Pancake, LIFE, 126
Okra and Tomatoes, Stewed, 138–39
olive oil, 5
omega-3 fats, 5, 19
omega-3 fish oils, 19
omelet:
  Broccoli & Cheese, 59
  Egg-Cellent Omelet with Vegetables &
    Cheese, 57
  Ham and Cheese Omelet with Chives,
    126
  Smoked Salmon, 214
  Stuffed Vegetable, 129
onions:
  Uncle Onion's Turkey Bean Chili, 222
  Turkey Sausage with Sautéed Peppers
    and Onions, 144
Open-Faced Tuna Melt, 130
Open-Faced Turkey Reuben, 130

orange:
LIFE Creamsicle Smoothie, 133
Orange Dijon Pork Tenderloin, 144
Orange Ginger Dressing, 62

pancakes:
Apple Cinnamon Pancakes with Yogurt
Topping, 124–25
LIFE Oatmeal, 126
LIFE Scallion Pancake with Sour Cream,
218
Panda Express, 211
Panera Bread, 207–208
parmesan:
Parmesan Broiled Tomato, 142
Tomato Parmesan Dressing, 62
parsnips, 22
partially hydrogenated oils, 5
pasta, 22
peanut butter, 25
peas, 22
Curried Chicken Salad with Sweet
Green Peas, 127
peer pressure, food, 287
Pelvic Bridges, 263
Peppers and Onions, Turkey Sausage with
Sautéed, 144
photographs, 9
Pita, Tuna Salad with, 58
Pita Pizza, Whole Wheat, 128
pizza:
Breakfast, 125
Whole Wheat Pita, 128
plateau, weight, 285–86
Popcorn Seasonings Blends, 134
pork:
Ham and Cheese Omelet with Chives,
126
Orange Dijon Pork Tenderloin, 144
Step One, 28, 292
Step Three, 160, 292
Step Two, 84, 292

portion sizes, 45–46, 286
restaurant, 238
Portobello Mushroom Caps, Stuffed, 227
posture, 259–60
potato, 22
chips, 25
Curry Sweet Potato Fries, 220
Sweet Potato Skillet, 124
poultry, 6
Step One, 27–28, 292
Step Three, 159, 292
Step Two, 83–84, 292
See also chicken; turkey
Power Arms, 258–59
preferences, food, 280
pre-plan meals, 7, 17
processed foods, 20
proteins, 5–6
breakfast substitutes, 85, 161
portion sizes, 45
Step One, 27–29, 47
swaps, 280
vegan, see vegan proteins
pudding, 75
Creamy Chocolate, 136
Creamy Vanilla, 136
Pumpkin Pudding, Vanilla, 57
Vanilla Pumpkin, 57
Pumpkin Pudding, Vanilla, 57
Puttanesca, Easy Chicken, 139

Quiche, LIFE, 137–38

Raspberry Vinaigrette, 61
recipes, 157
Step One, 57–69
Step Three, 213–28
Step Two, 119–44
See also menus and recipes; specific
recipes
recreation. See exercise

relationships, 3, 245–46
Relearn. *See* Step Two (Relearn)
Release. *See* Step One (Release)
reminders, weight loss, 286
Reshape. *See* Step Three (Reshape)
resistance training, 267–72, 285
    tips, 268
restaurants, 151, 282
    portion sizes, 238
    Step One options, 56
    Step Three options, 202–213
    Step Two options, 116–19
Reuben, Open-Faced Turkey, 130
rewards, 230, 242
rice, 22
Rosemary Granita, Grapefruit, 135
Rosner, Mary, 149–50, 229–30
running, 256
Russell, Penny, 145–46

salad, 150
    Chicken, 217
    Chicken-Apple Salad Chop, 128
    Crab, 215
    Curried Chicken Salad with Sweet
        Green Peas, 127
    Egg White, 215
    Greek Salad with Feta, 217
    LIFE Dinner Salad, 59–60
    Sicilian Tuna, 216
    Tuna Salad with Pita, 58–59
    Veggie Tuna, 127
salmon:
    Easy Cheesy Salmon Melt, 216
    Ginger Lime Salmon Cakes, 224
    Microwave Poached Salmon with Lemon
        Dill Sauce, 219
    Salmon Teriyaki, 66
    Smoked Salmon Omelet, 214
salt, 20
salty alternatives, 284
saturated fats, 5

Sausage with Sautéed Peppers and Onions,
    Turkey, 144
Sautéed Spinach, 65
Savory Almonds, 133
Scallion Pancake with Sour Cream, LIFE,
    218
schedule, eating on a, 17
seafood. *See* fish and seafood
seasonings, 34
    Step One, 34–36, 300–301
    Step Three, 167–70, 301
    Step Two, 91–93, 301
Seated Reverse Fly, 271–72
Seated Rows, 271
self-confidence, 3
serving sizes, appropriate, 45–46, 286
Shepherd's Pie, LIFE, 143
shrimp:
    Chesapeake Shrimp Boil, 138
    Lemon Garlic Shrimp, 224
    Shrimp Ceviche with Lime, 142
Sicilian Tuna Salad, 216
Side-to-Side Lunges, 270
sleep, 3, 286
Sloppy Joes, Chicken, 225
Smoked Salmon Omelet, 214
smoothie:
    LIFE Banana Cardamom, 132
    LIFE Blueberry Mango, 132
    LIFE Creamsicle, 133
    LIFE Strawberry Banana, 132–33
snacks. *See* afternoon snack; LIFE Healthy
        Extras; nighttime snack
soft drinks, diet, 20, 23
Sorbet, Blueberry Mango, 135
soup, 150
    LIFE Veggie, 63–65
    Minestrone, 131
Sour Cream, LIFE Scallion Pancake with,
    218
soy, 47
Speed Play, 261, 266
Spice Muffins, LIFE Carrot, 121

spinach:
  Sautéed, 65
  Spinach and Feta Egg Scramble, 214
Starbucks, 209
starches, 20, 22, 150
  portions sizes, 46
  Step Three, 164
  Step Two, 88
Step Four (Reveal), 6, 231–42
  eating to maintain weight loss, 231–32
  enjoying your success, 238–39
  exercise, 273–74
  food rules: dos and don'ts, 232–33
  LIFE Healthy Extras, 237–38
Stephenson, Tammy, 252–53
Step One (Release), 6, 15–72, 286
  advice for success, 17
  afternoon snack, 21, 38–40, 303–304
  beverages, 37–38, 41, 302, 306
  breakfast, 21, 26–34, 48–56, 57–58
  days one through seven, 48–55
  dinner, 21, 26–34, 48–56, 59–69
  Easiest Meals At-A-Glance, 55
  exercise, 254–60
  food allowed at meals, 26–34, 292–306
  food rules: dos and don'ts, 20–23
  lunch, 21, 26–34, 38–46, 58–59
  menus and recipes, 47–69
  restaurant options, 56
  seasonings, condiments, marinades, and
    fats, 34–36, 300–301
  serving sizes, 45–46
  supplements, 17–19
  Unlimited Foods, 41–42, 306
Step Three (Reshape), 6, 149–230
  afternoon snack, 153, 170–73, 179–99,
    305
  beverages, 170, 174, 302, 306
  breakfast, 153, 158–67, 179–89, 202,
    213–14
  days one through twenty-one, 179–99
  dinner, 153, 158–67, 179–99, 203–204
  Easiest Meals At-A-Glance, 200–201

  exercise, 266–72
  fast food options, 204–213
  food allowed at meals, 158–67, 292–306
  food rules: dos and don'ts, 152–54
  LIFE Healthy Extras, 151, 152
  lunch, 153, 158–67, 179–99, 202–203,
    215–18
  menus and recipes, 177–228
  restaurant options, 202–213
  rules, 150–51
  seasonings, condiments, marinades, and
    healthy fats, 167–70, 300–301
  Unlimited Foods, 174, 306
Step Two (Relearn), 6, 73–147
  afternoon snack, 78, 94–96, 101–114,
    304
  beverages, 94, 96–97, 132–37, 302, 306
  breakfast, 78, 82–91, 101–115, 117
  day one through fourteen, 101–114
  dinner, 78, 82–91, 101–115, 118–19,
    137–44
  Easiest Meals At-A-Glance, 115–16
  exercise, 260–66
  food allowed at meals, 82–91, 292–306
  food rules: dos and don'ts, 76–77
  fun foods, 132–37
  LIFE Healthy Extras, 75–76
  lunch, 78, 82–91, 101–115, 117–18,
    127–31
  menus and recipes, 100–144
  restaurant options, 116–19
  rules, 74
  seasonings, condiments, marinades, and
    healthy fats, 91–93, 300–301
  Unlimited Foods, 96–97, 306
Stewed Okra and Tomatoes, 138–39
Strawberry Banana Smoothie, LIFE,
  132–33
strength and stamina, 3
stress, 8, 250
Stuffed Portobello Mushroom Caps, 227
Stuffed Vegetable Omelet, 129
Subway, 208–209

success:
    advice for, 17
    enjoying your, 238–39
    secrets for, 6–8
sugar, 16, 20
    substitutes, 20, 23, 74
sugarless gum, 40
Summer Mint Tea, 41
Sumo Squats, 269
supplements, 17–19
Sweet and Sour Chicken, 228
Sweet Green Peas, Curried Chicken Salad
    with, 127
sweet potato:
    Curry Sweet Potato Fries, 220
    Sweet Potato Skillet, 124
sweet treats, 283

Taco Bell, 209
Tacos, Turkey, 227
Tandoori Halibut Kebabs, 141
Tea, Summer Mint, 41
television, and eating, 8
teriyaki:
    Beef, 65–66
    Chicken, 67
    Salmon, 65
    Tofu, 67–68
Thousand Island Dressing, 61
Tidwell, Mandy, 234–36
tofu, 47
    Tofu Teriyaki, 67–68
tomato:
    Parmesan Broiled Tomato, 142
    Stewed Okra and Tomatoes, 138
    Tomato Parmesan Dressing, 62
Tortilla Roll Up, Turkey, 129
trans fats, 5
travel, 282
trigger foods, avoiding, 6–7, 25
tuna:
    Open-Faced Tuna Melt, 130

Sicilian Tuna Salad, 216
Tuna Salad with Pita, 58–59
Veggie Tuna Salad, 127
turkey:
    Cheddar Turkey Burger with Sautéed
        Mushrooms, 68
    E-Z Turkey Burger, 68
    Mini Turkey Meatloaves, 221
    Open-Faced Turkey Reuben, 130
    Turkey Sausage with Sautéed Peppers
        and Onions, 144
    Turkey Tacos, 227
    Turkey Tortilla Roll Up, 129
    Uncle Onion's Turkey Bean Chili, 222
    See also poultry

Uncle Onion's Turkey Bean Chili, 222
unhealthy foods, getting rid of, 7
Unlimited Foods, 7, 17, 20, 34, 91, 282–83
    Step One, 41–42, 306
    Step Three, 174, 306
    Step Two, 96–97, 306

vanilla:
    Creamy Vanilla Pudding, 136
    Vanilla French Toast, 213–14
    Vanilla Pumpkin Pudding, 57
vegan proteins, 47
    Step One, 29, 294
    Step Three, 161–62, 294
    Step Two, 85, 294
    See also specific foods
vegetables, 5
    afternoon snack, 172–73, 305
    cost of, 281
    Egg-Cellent Omelet with Vegetables &
        Cheese, 57
    Fish Fillet en Papillote with Garden
        Vegetables, 223
    LIFE Veggie Soup, 63–65
    Loaded Veggie Frittata, 226

Step One, 29–31, 41, 295–96
Step Three, 162–64, 172–73, 296
Step Two, 85–88, 296
Stuffed Vegetable Omelet, 129
Veggie Tuna Salad, 127
See also specific vegetables
vegetarians, 47, 100, 177
vinaigrette:
    Balsamic, 60
    Raspberry, 61
vinegar, 34
vitamins and minerals, 5, 17–19
    calcium, 18
    D, 18
    multivitamin, 18
    supplements, 17–19

walking, 254–60
    guidelines, 256–60, 261
Walking Into Walls, 264

Walnut Stuffed Chicken Breast,
    Gorgonzola-, 225–26
water, 20
    calorie–free naturally flavored, 38
weight loss, eating to maintain, 231–32
weight plateau, breaking through, 285–86
Wendy's, 206–207
Wheaton, Sherry, 145–46
whole grains, 5
    Step One, 31–32, 297
    Step Three, 164–65, 297
    Step Two, 88–89, 297
Whole Wheat Pita Pizza, 128
wine, 22
women, 47, 100, 177

yogurt, 75
    afternoon snack, 39, 95, 171, 303–305
    Apple Cinnamon Pancakes with Yogurt
        Topping, 124–25